Overcoming Common Problems

Everything Your GP Doesn't Have Time to Tell You About Arthritis

DR MATT PICCAVER

sheldon **PRESS**

First published in Great Britain in 2017

Sheldon Press
36 Causton Street
London SW1P 4ST
www.sheldonpress.co.uk

British Library Cataloguing-in-Publication Data
A catalogue record for this book is available from the British Library

ISBN 978-1-84709-463-6
eBook ISBN 978-1-84709-464-3

Typeset by Fakenham Prepress Solutions, Fakenham, Norfolk NR21 8NN
First printed in Great Britain by Ashford Colour Press
Subsequently digitally printed in Great Britain

eBook by Fakenham Prepress Solutions, Fakenham, Norfolk NR21 8NN

Produced on paper from sustainable forests

This book is dedicated to my super-tolerant wife, my children, my family at large. It is also dedicated to my teachers, colleagues and patients. (My wife tells me that's basically everyone I know. She has a point.)

Contents

Note to the reader

This is not a medical book and is not intended to replace advice from your doctor. Consult your pharmacist or doctor if you believe you have any of the symptoms described, and if you think you might need medical help.

Introduction

Sometimes I think aching is normal. The older I get, the more I tend to hurt. Somewhere. It might be that funny twinge I get when I turn my head to the right and look up a bit. That sort of electric shock pain that for a split second reminds me I have a neck and a head. Most of the time our body parts merrily sit there, silently doing their jobs, until one day they go wrong. Hopefully not very wrong, hopefully with a bit of warning, and hopefully nothing too final.

Our bodies are not too bad at telling us when something is wrong. They're not great, but on the whole they are reasonably effective at alerting us when something is amiss. Probably one of the most common reasons for coming to see a doctor is pain. Pain is a great way of telling us something *might* be wrong. I say *might* as for some of us pain continues, even if the original noxious stimulus has long gone. I see countless people with joint pain, and that is what this book is about.

If we're lucky, we get old. One day at a time, a little older, possibly wiser, and probably a little more worn out. Aging brings with it many things, including some unwelcome guests that are hard to shift. Life etches itself upon us, indelibly. We pick up the telltale signs of everyday encounters. Every injury tells a story. Every scar is a badge of experience, a bit like the medals proudly worn by an old soldier.

I still can't feel my right little toe. One day in the gym, as a newly qualified doctor, I felt something go pop. For those of you in the know, I was doing a dorsal raise. You lie on your front and lift your head and chest off the ground. Regardless, something went ping, I developed pain down the back of my right leg that lasted for a while, then settled. But even to this day, if I lift something awkwardly or sit in a certain position, the pain comes back. I know I have a little toe. I can't say it seems to do much and if it wasn't there I'm not certain I'd miss it.

My left knee still aches from time to time. My medial meniscus, apparently. This is the inner part of the knee lined with cartilage, which is a lubricating tissue that stops bone rubbing on bone. It's the gristly bit on the end of a chicken leg, except in us it's much bigger. I told the orthopaedic surgeon that it was a 'sporting injury'. In reality the injury happened during a choreographed lightsaber duel that my friend and I thought was hilarious. There might have been alcohol involved. I'm pretty sure it was a fancy-dress party. I think my friend's a paediatrician now and as far as I know he has survived unscathed.

We all have hobbies or jobs that over time take their toll. I don't meet many manual workers who don't ache somewhere by the time they hit their mid-fifties, many typists of yesteryear without arthritis of their hands and shoulders (usually their right), or ex-footballers without dodgy knees.

This book is for all of us who creak, grind and crack when we move. Who might have joints that swell in the mornings or become hot and red and angry. It's for those of us who might drop something and have to consider carefully whether or not to pick it up. It's for those of us who make that funny noise when we sit down. A sort of groaning sigh. You know the one.

This book is for those of us who are no strangers to throbbing, shooting or burning pain. Pain that came a long time ago and stayed for good. Pain that comes when you move or stays when you stop. Pain that's there when you wake up and when you go to sleep. Pain that wakes you in the night or stops you in your tracks.

This is the book for those with stiff joints. Joints that are told to do one thing, yet have a mind of their own. Joints that once helped you play a sport or hold down a job, but now just let you down.

This is the book for those of us made 'bionic', receiving new joints in place of old. Those of us who are now a little bit machine.

As a GP I have ten minutes to help you. Ten minutes to find out what's wrong, make a diagnosis, come up with a treatment and explain to you everything you need to know about your disease.

Sometimes it can take half that time just to take your coat off. This is the book for those of us who leave our doctor's room thinking 'What did he/she say?' There is a fair amount of research to suggest that, many times, people don't really remember much about what their doctor has told them. Perhaps a couple of facts – usually about the diagnosis rather than the treatment. Now and again I'll receive a call or message advising me that 'Mrs X has forgotten what you told her', or 'When does Mr Y need to get his X-ray again?'

I've realized that I probably spend much of my time saying the same things to different people. The diagnosis, treatment, side effects of medicines and what happens next. It's clear that I can't possibly tell people everything they need to know in the time we have together. We have to pick and choose, and hope that, between the patient and the doctor, we both have roughly the same recollection of the consultation. In my experience, this almost never happens, which is why we keep meticulous notes. Over the course of a year, I probably have anywhere up to ten thousand consultations. Some people I might see repeatedly; others just once. I work in a general practice, I work in out-of-hours clinics seeing urgent cases and in extended hours clinics. Consequently, I find it hard to remember much between appointments and have to make good notes as an aide memoire.

I tend to write many things down for my patients, usually in the form of bullet points. Get this test done, take these tablets, see me in so many weeks and watch out for so and so. The name changes, the advice varies a little, adjusted according to the patient to some degree. Over the years of practice, I've probably written enough information for patients to fill a book, so I thought I'd write one.

This book is everything your GP doesn't have time to tell you about arthritis: symptoms, diagnosis and treatment options. A bit of science and a lot of information about how you can help yourself and when to get help. We'll find out what arthritis is, the different types of arthritis there are and how they can affect us. We'll develop a greater understanding of how our bodies work. We'll delve into the science of how our joints work and what happens when they don't. We'll talk about the treatments available, either over the counter or from your doctor. We'll find out about the process, what happens from when you see your doctor to the steps involved in your treatment. We'll hear from people who have arthritis and how they live their lives with the condition, rather than suffer from it. We'll find out about what we can do to help ourselves and what hopes we have for the future regarding the treatment of arthritis.

1

What is arthritis?

'Arthritis' is a general term referring to a disease of the joints. Medical terminology is essentially a description of the ailment, usually translated from Latin, Greek or a mixture of the two, but, more often than not, the name tells us what the ailment is. *Arthron* is Greek for 'joints' and *-itis* refers to inflammation. You'll hear *-itis* at the end of many names for diseases. Tonsillitis, appendicitis, colitis – in these cases inflammation of the tonsils, appendix and colon, and the large bowel. This book is about joints, so we'll leave the other bits to one side for the time being.

Arthritis takes a variety of different forms and has a number of different causes. To truly understand the condition, we need to know a little more about how we are put together. For many people I meet, the workings of the body are a mystery. This is a little like the way I view my car. I know where to put the fuel. I know where the exhaust is. I have a vague idea about how to check the oil and when to change the tyres. Outside that, it is a complete mystery. When I visit my mechanic he makes it seem easy. I take my car, bits get replaced, I pay the bill and it seems to work better. My dad, however, appears to have this in-built knowledge of how all things mechanical seem to work. A little noise or slight change in the way his car handles and he is on it like a shot. He's handy with a spanner and can usually fix most problems. People perhaps aren't so readily fixed, but with a little knowledge, we can understand more how our body works, what happens when it goes wrong and how to help ourselves fix it (if we can).

Joints are a junction between bones. There are 206 bones in the human skeleton. These bones offer a compromise between protection, movement and structure. They give our body form, protect major organs, offer points of attachment for muscles and allow us to move. Solid enough to protect us from injury (to some degree), but light enough to allow us to traverse the Earth. To me, the human body is a marvel of biological engineering; a perfect example of balance between form and function.

There are hundreds of different joints in the human body, which are categorized by type. Each type serves a different purpose. Joints may stick one bone to another, they might allow a little give or a free range of movement.

Fibrous joints are those that stick bits of bone to other bits of bone. By and large, there shouldn't be much movement in these. They include the joints (called sutures) between the plates of the skull. When we're born, the bones that make up the skull are not joined; hence the 'soft spot' we often notice on the top of a baby's head. This is called the anterior fontanelle. If our skull bones were fused together in the womb, childbirth would be even more difficult and painful than it already is. These bones overlap and allow the baby's head to reduce in size during labour. During the early stages of life, they fuse to provide the protective solid casing of the skull.

Cartilaginous joints are those that are lined with cartilage; hence the name. If you've ever had a chicken leg (with apologies to my vegetarian friends), you'll have noticed the soft, white material on the ends of the bone. This is cartilage. There are three types of cartilage, called hyaline, elastic and fibrocartilage. The latter is the most abundant and found in a few joints such as the jaw bone (temporomandibular joint), between the collarbone and breastbone (sternoclavicular joint) and some of the joints between the ribs and breastbone (sternochondral joints). Hyaline is also found in a joint between the top of the shoulder blade and the collar bone, called the acromioclavicular joint. This is often a site of wear, delightfully called 'degenerative change', and is the slightly bumpy bit just beneath where a bra strap sits on the shoulder (should you be inclined to wear one). These joints belong to a class of joint called atypical synovial joints. They're atypical because they are different from the 'typical' synovial joint. They don't perform the function that the synovial joints are mainly known for, which is movement. The atypical joints are somewhere in-between the fixed ones, such as those that join the plates of our skulls together and the ones that move a lot, such as elbows, knees, hips and so on. They move – a bit. When we move our shoulders, the acromioclavicular joint moves a little. It helps contribute to the freedom of movement that we have in our shoulders. If you want to know what happens when that joint is stiff or inflamed, try moving your arm while someone presses down on your shoulder. The movement is OK, but it isn't anywhere near as good as when the hand is taken off it.

If you want to know what the joints between some of the ribs and the breastbone do, try breathing in deeply while someone gives you a bear hug (gently, however – I will accept no responsibility for injuries caused during this experiment). Again, you will find that you can breathe in a bit, but can't quite get the big lungful you might need when exerting yourself. These joints provide a bit of give, a little movement, but aren't really there to provide the bulk of your mobility. You notice when they don't work so well, however.

The rest of the joints are the ones we tend to notice when we suffer from arthritis. They are called synovial joints. These joints are lined with the shiny stuff called hyaline cartilage. They're enclosed in a capsule lined with synovium, a tissue that produces synovial fluid. The whole joint is lined with synovium except where cartilage is present. Imagine it as a sack containing a little lubrication. These joints, rather than being bone-on-bone (or, rather, cartilage-on-cartilage), are separated by a thin layer of fluid. This fluid is made by cells within the synovium. A normal healthy knee can have around 2 ml of synovial fluid. In some respects we've all got a little 'water on the knee'.

Now, 'I'm a doctor, Jim, not an engineer', but there are such things as 'self-lubricating ball joints'. These are joints that can be found in types of suspension in cars and they lubricate themselves internally, much like our synovial joints. Nature has beaten the engineers to it.

Synovial fluid is truly amazing stuff – much more complex than water. It behaves like something called a non-Newtonian fluid. (I told you there would be science.) Non-Newtonian fluids are fascinating things. Unlike water, non-Newtonian fluids increase their viscosity when under stress. They get sort of thicker, more gloopy, so when the fluid in the joint is under pressure, such as when running, the fluid becomes thicker, helping provide something of a cushioning effect, at least in theory.

When I was younger, I once watched an experiment in which a swimming pool was filled with custard. The presenter set out to prove that you can run on the surface of a fluid. He set out at a fast pace, easily covering the bright yellow surface of the swimming pool. That is until he stopped. At which point he sank. By walking quickly, he placed the fluid under pressure and it kept him buoyant. When he stopped, the fluid became less gloopy, more liquid, and down he went. Then they tried to pull him out and the fluid tightened its grip.

The moral of this story: synovial fluid is a bit like custard. Sort of. It gets viscous when it is under pressure, cushioning the joints when they are under load, then eases up when the pressure is taken off.

The joints that tend to develop arthritis (or at least the ones we tend to notice) are the load-bearing joints, particularly the hips and knees. These tend to be the ones that bother us the most and therefore the ones which get replaced. That said, arthritis can affect any synovial joint.

We can further divide these synovial joints into different types, depending on their function. Let us start, in no particular order, with the hands. As I type, I can see the joints in my fingers working. These are called hinge joints. They do exactly what you would expect from this descriptive name. There is a bone on either side of each joint and the joint is lined with cartilage and a little of the lubricating synovial fluid we discussed earlier, which allows each finger to bend as required. The joints work just like a hinge on a door.

In case you hadn't guessed, I find people and the human body fascinating and the hands are amazing parts of our bodies. Starting from the tips, we have the phalanges – three in each finger, two in the thumb. These are the small bones that make up the fingers. The joints between the phalanges take a real battering throughout life and can be affected by rheumatoid and osteoarthritis alike (more on those later). Our hands allow us to carry out delicate procedures, such as threading a needle or holding a pen. They can provide us with amazing strength. Next time you see a rock climber, watch his or her fingers. I've seen many an example of people clinging on with only one or two fingers. The finger joints are delicate, strong and durable.

The joints between the phalanges are called interphalangeal joints, and are often a site of arthritis. Working up the hand, we meet the metacarpals. These are a series of long bones joining the phalanges to the carpal bones. They provide the bulk of the structure of the palm of the hand. The joints between the phalanges and the metacarpals are called metacarpophalangeal joints. They're different from the hinge joints of the fingers and called condyloid joints. They too work like a hinge, but the surface is curved. Take a look at your hand and notice how, when you make a fist, there is a much greater range of movement at the knuckle (the metacarpophalangeal joints) than between the bones of the fingers. The curved surface of the joint allows us to curl our fingers palm-wards.

Further up the hand towards the wrist, we meet the carpals. These are a group of eight small bones between the metacarpals and wrist. They give form to the lower part of the palm of the hand, providing a little movement, but largely structure, to our hands. These joints slide against each other. They aren't there to provide the sorts of movements we get at the hip or shoulder, or even our fingers, but imagine trying to catch a ball with a perfectly flat palm. Chances are you wouldn't be very successful, and it would probably be rather painful too.

Working up the arm, we reach the wrist joint. This is another synovial joint, between the carpals and the main bone in the forearm, called the ulnar. Take a look at your wrist and move it about. Make a fist and curl it towards you. This is called flexion, and you can see our wrists have a good range of movement in terms of flexion. Cock the wrist back, and this is extension. Slightly less movement again, but still good. We can move our wrists from side to side, but not as much as we can flex or extend. This provides stability in lateral movement (side to side) and flexibility in flexion and extension.

Further up the arm, we meet the elbow. The elbow is a hinge joint, between the bones in the lower arm and the large bone in the upper arm, called the humerus (hence its other name, the 'funny bone'). It provides a great range of movement in one plane, namely flexion and extension. It doesn't have much give from side to side.

Higher up and we have the shoulder joint. The shoulder is a ball-and-socket joint. If you want to see how great a range of movement the shoulder has, watch a bowler in a cricket match. As a bit of a sacrifice for the sake of this wide range of movement, the shoulder has a very shallow socket and thus is held in place by the muscle bulk of the shoulder. Consequently, some people may dislocate their shoulder with greater ease than would be the case with the other joints.

On our tour of the joints of the body, let us move to the spine. The spine needs to provide protection for the spinal cord, flexibility, a site for connection of muscles and bones and permit us to walk upright. It consists of bones called vertebrae and discs between them called intervertebral discs. The vertebrae are almost like a stack of building blocks, but in each part of the spine, their shape is a little different from those elsewhere. In general, they have spaces in the middle, to allow the spinal cord to pass through, and gaps either side to allow nerves to branch off around the body. They have joints called facet joints that allow each one to articulate with the bone beneath it. Facet joints are a type of joint called a plane joint. They allow each half of the joint to slide, giving movement in one plane, hence the name.

Starting at the top, the vertebrae of the neck are called cervical vertebrae. 'Cervical' refers to neck, hence the term cervix referring to the neck of the womb. Cervical vertebrae are small, flat, round discs with, again, space for the spinal cord. They're much thinner than the vertebrae further down the spine as the load they carry is largely that of the head. Much like a certain circular mint with a hole in the middle, they are, in essence, discs of bone that allow the spinal cord to pass through them. They move together in such a way as to provide a high level of mobility, allowing a large range of movement at the neck. Left, right, up, down, side to side – but not behind. We've sacrificed complete freedom of movement in order to keep the head pointing forward.

The next vertebrae down are the thoracic vertebrae. They permit forward flexion more than rotation, and also join to our ribs. Further down, we have the lumbar vertebrae – large, strong load-bearing vertebrae that have to support the weight of the entire upper body. They are the biggest of the vertebrae for this very reason. Finally, we have the sacral vertebrae. These are fused to make a large triangular bone (the sacrum) that forms the back of the pelvis. At the bottom is the coccyx, the little bone vestige of a tail, again fused like the sacrum.

In total, there are 33 vertebrae: 7 cervical, 12 thoracic, 5 lumbar, 5 sacral and 4 in the coccyx. These 33 bones give us the primary scaffold for our limbs.

Further south is the pelvis, joined by very strong ligaments to the sacrum, and each side is a hip joint. The pelvis protects vital internal organs as well as forming the foundations of our legs.

The hip joints, like the shoulders, are ball-and-socket joints. Unlike the shoulders, though, the hip joints each consist of a deep socket, called the acetabulum. It encloses a large portion of the head of the thigh bone (the femur), so is a much more stable joint than the shoulder. It is harder to dislocate, but the range of movement is less than the shoulder. You can't scratch your back with your foot (usually), whereas you can with your hand.

We work our way down to the knees, which consist of another type of hinge joint, and are often a site of osteoarthritis. The knees take a real beating over a lifetime. It is estimated that our knee joints experience two to three times our body weight when we walk, and three to four times our body weight when we run. Is it any wonder they may eventually need to be replaced in time? We stand anywhere from about nine months of age and a great deal for the rest of our lives.

Working down, we come to the ankle joint – another type of hinge joint, made up of the end of the shin bone (the tibia) and the talus, which sits on top of the heel bone, called the calcaneum. Then, moving to the feet, there are the tarsal bones, metatarsals and some more phalanges. While there are similarities between the feet and the hands, the feet have evolved to carry us and our body weight. Each foot, to some extent, is like a dome or bridge, with a long arch running from toe to heel, and a shorter one from side to side. Feet provide stability and support, but generally do not have a whole lot of dexterity. Most of us tend not to write with our feet, but there are lots of people who do, perhaps as a result of an injury or disability. Like the other joints of the lower limbs, the joints of the feet withstand constant use and considerable load.

If we take a look at our hands again, we notice that we are more than just bones. Our joints consist of ligaments, tendons and muscles. Ligaments join bone to bone and can be found in many places in the body. We have probably all heard of cases of footballers especially injuring their cruciate ligaments. These are ligaments found in the knee that join the thigh bone to the shin bone and add stability to the joint. They can be readily injured in high-impact sports, such as football, often during a twisting injury. The foot stays planted, but the thigh bone twists and snap goes the ligament.

We also have the tendons. Tendons join muscles to bones. Perhaps the most widely known tendon is the Achilles tendon. This anchors the calf muscle to the heel bone, and allows you to push your foot downwards. Every time you accelerate or depress the clutch in the car, you're using your Achilles tendon. Named after the ancient Greek hero Achilles, said to have been dipped in the River Styx by his mother to render him invulnerable. Unfortunately, she held him by the heel and this one point was his only weak spot, which ultimately was his undoing. Achilles was killed by a poisoned arrow by Paris during the Trojan War.

Our own Achilles tendons are vulnerable too and it is possible to tear or rupture them. I've known many people feel their tendons snap, often during sport. Sports requiring sudden explosive movements from a standstill, especially if we've not warmed up or have been away from a sport for a while, can cause the Achilles tendon to go ping.

There are a number of different types of arthritis, as well as other causes of joint pain and swelling. The majority of this book is about two types of arthritis: osteoarthritis – 'wear and tear arthritis' – and inflammatory arthritis, with rheumatoid arthritis being a member of this family of diseases. The next chapter is about the sort of arthritis that many of us can expect to develop, particularly as we get older – namely, osteoarthritis.

2

Osteoarthritis

Osteoarthritis is really, really common. If I think hard enough, I suspect I'll see someone with potential osteoarthritis in every surgery. In fact, the World Health Organization (WHO) ranks diseases of the muscles, bones or joints as the most common reasons for seeing your GP.

According to the charity Arthritis Research UK, nearly nine million people in the UK have sought treatment for osteoarthritis. The WHO estimates that around 21 per cent of the UK population is undergoing treatment for some form of long-term muscle or joint issue, of which osteoarthritis makes up a considerable proportion. Across the globe, around 10 per cent of men and 20 per cent of women will have some degree of osteoarthritis that is significant enough to cause them various degrees of difficulty. Of those with osteoarthritis, 80 per cent of people will have some degree of limitation of movement. About a quarter of people with arthritis may find that it is bad enough to stop them carrying out their normal daily activities. This might be washing, dressing or walking short distances, for example. Across the globe, it is one of the leading causes of disability.

Osteoarthritis is largely a disease of aging, which means many of us will become all too familiar with it if we aren't already. The older we get, the more likely we are to develop osteoarthritis. About a third of people in the UK over the age of 45 years are thought to have osteoarthritis. This number rises as we pass the age of 75, to about half of all women and about 40 per cent of men (according to Arthritis Research UK, men tend to go to their doctors a little less with arthritis than do women).

Diane
I had a chat with Diane, who kindly allowed me to share her story. Diane is a former district nurse in her fifties. She's given her life to the care of others, and used to play a lot of sport. Arthritis runs in her family, and she started getting problems in her mid-forties.

'It all just came at once,' she told me.

When she first started having problems, she went to see her GP. 'My GP was superb,' she told me. Referred up to a consultant orthopaedic surgeon, she has gone on to have several joint replacements and is currently waiting for a shoulder replacement.

Prior to her surgery, she'd 'never known pain like it'. By the time of her operation, her cartilage had worn to such an extent that her joints were bone on bone.

No stranger to surgery by now, Diane has never had a bad experience. 'I was in theatre within an hour of getting to hospital' she said.

She still needs pain relief, however.

'I take meloxicam, paracetamol, morphine both tablet and liquid, and amitriptyline'. These cross the full range of anti-inflammatory, opioid and neuropathic agents we will talk about later.

I asked her what else helps her joints.

'I bought a hot tub. It helps a great deal.'

I asked her what advice she had for anyone else suffering from osteoarthritis.

'Watch your weight and keep mobile.'

It's pretty clear that osteoarthritis is a big deal. Potentially the most common reason for coming to see someone like me, it is something that may greet many of us as we age.

While many joints may be affected by osteoarthritis, the joints most commonly affected are the hip, knee, foot, ankle and wrist. This is probably no surprise. The joints of the lower limbs are subject to considerable load. They must support and convey us from the day we learn to walk to the day we die. Wrist joints, again, are sites of load, but perhaps in different ways from the joints in our legs. We might not put our full body weight through our wrists, but all jobs or hobbies involve our wrist joints at some point. I frequently meet people with shoulder and hand arthritis too.

When I first started at medical school, one of the earliest lectures I can recall taught me about the different areas of study that awaited us. We had biochemistry, the study of the complex chemical reactions and interactions that go on in our bodies. Almost like zooming in to a map, we'd study the human body at the level of molecules, cells, tissues, organ systems and the body as a whole. I'm going to outline the different processes and problems that occur in osteoarthritis. Here comes another science bit.

Many of us refer to osteoarthritis as 'wear and tear' arthritis, thinking parts of us gradually wear out much like bits of our cars might do. Perhaps unsurprisingly, it is a little more complex than that. The exact mechanism behind the development of osteoarthritis has been and continues to be the subject of a great deal of study. If a chemical process causing osteoarthritis to occur can be found, then perhaps medications or treatments can be developed to target and potentially cure osteoarthritis. Perhaps one day 'wear and tear' arthritis won't be an inevitable part of life.

One of the most common sites of osteoarthritis is the knee joint, so perhaps it makes sense to talk about how arthritis develops in the context of this joint. You may recall from earlier on that I once injured my knee, the cartilage in particular. Leaping around, beered up and laughing, I landed on my left knee and, when I stood up, I immediately felt pain on the inner aspect of that knee. Thankfully, I was sufficiently socially anaesthetized that the pain was kept to a minimum. The following day, though, I felt pain, especially when walking. My knee felt a bit stiff as well and there was a little swelling. Once the swelling had settled down, I began to notice that I had to throw my leg forwards to get it to straighten properly. This is called locking. Over time it improved, but it still happens occasionally. In time, I anticipate I'll develop osteoarthritis in that knee and perhaps the other one too.

As mentioned above the mechanism behind the development of osteoarthritis is the subject of extensive research and theories have evolved from it being due to wear and tear to a much more complex process being involved. There are a number of areas of research at the moment.

Ligament damage may occur. This might be to the cruciates or the collateral ligaments in the case of the knee. Ligaments provide stability and keep the knee joint aligned. Muscles may become weak, perhaps as a result of underuse, injury or general atrophy due to aging. These may also lead to an element of instability or loss of joint alignment. This contributes to increased load (as does being overweight in my case), which then causes what's referred to as 'microtrauma' in and around the joint. Certain occupations can cause considerable load in the joint too. Inflammation then occurs. Inflammation is the body's way of dealing with something it doesn't like as well as its attempt to heal itself. There might be increased fluid in the knee and inflammation of the synovium (the bag in which the knee joint sits). A number of biochemical processes have also been associated with the development of osteoarthritis with exotic-sounding names such as tumour necrosis factor alpha, metalloproteinases and interleukins, to name but a few. They are associated with inflammation and are the subject of considerable research interest. Perhaps one day we will truly understand the mechanism behind the development of osteoarthritis and therefore be in a position to develop effective treatments.

There are changes to the bone. Inflammation occurs beneath the cartilage. In X-rays we might see the development of cysts and scarring of the bone. We also see extra bone, called osteophytes – small extra spurs of bone around the affected joint. Whether they cause a problem or not is subject to debate, but they're seen fairly commonly in joint X-rays and help us decide on a diagnosis.

In my knee, I suspect I developed cartilage damage. This has caused a little change in the mechanics of the movement of my knee. In time, if not already, I'll develop the microtrauma – tiny injuries to the knee – mentioned above. This may lead to or involve an inflammatory process, leading to pain and the development of osteoarthritis. In time, at least, if not presently.

There is something a little depressing about knowing your potential fate and this is the case for me, at least as far as my knees are concerned. One of the perils of medical training is an all too real insight into the frailties of our physical form and being able to detect hints of what the future may hold.

I spoke to Tonia Vincent, Professor of Musculoskeletal Biology at the University of Oxford. While 'wear and tear' is now an inaccurate description of osteoarthritis, it's still one she uses in clinic as it's readily understandable by patients. 'Patients find it easy to understand,' she said. Of the particular things we discussed, one thing of interest is how cartilage responds to mechanical load – the everyday demands that we put on our joints.

Chondrocytes are the cells that make cartilage. The way they respond to load or injury in the joint may be implicated in the development of osteoarthritis. In the case of damage to the cartilage, a remodelling response occurs. Over time, remodelling of the cartilage ultimately leads to weakness. It is not 'wear' as such, more inadequate repair – or, more accurately, imperfect repair. The cartilage is remodelled with the help of a number of enzymes grouped together, called aggrecanases.

Professor Vincent advised that there are three important things to consider in the context of the development of osteoarthritis. The first is mechanical load. As noted earlier, joints are subject to load in some form most of the time, and there is some evidence to suggest that chondrocytes can make the building blocks of cartilage in the event of injury, but this building block (collagen) isn't integrated into the cartilage very well. A little wear and an attempt at repair.

The second important factor that may be involved in developing osteoarthritis is the mechanics of movement. As we get older, our ability to 'mechano-protect' diminishes. Every action we carry out results in a very rapid set of processes that protect our joints and reduce the load and potential damage through them. As we age, however, these mechanisms become less effective. Here comes another car analogy. Modern cars are designed to protect passengers in the event of an accident. Seat belt pre-tensioners fire off before impact, causing the seat belt to tighten a split second before we crash. If this didn't happen, we'd still be kept in our seats, but the forces through our bodies might be greater. As we age, the protective mechanisms that reduce the forces through our joints do not work as well as they did when we were younger, contributing to the development of osteoarthritis. Cartilage is an active tissue. Rather than just an inert shiny surface, it is filled with cells and can deteriorate over time, particularly if underused.

'If you imagine Tim Peake in space,' explained Professor Vincent, 'his cartilage would have diminished through disuse after six months in orbit.'

We might not be spending much time in orbit ourselves, but if you imagine being immobilized for some time, the quality of your cartilage will reduce. This might happen after a prolonged stay in hospital or after having a leg in a cast.

The other important point Professor Vincent made is about the biochemical messages occurring in the development of osteoarthritis. What happens in a joint that means these attempts at healing aren't quite as successful as we'd hope? In experiments with dogs, it has been shown that cartilage can redevelop in joints where there has been previous cartilage loss (usually by putting the dog's leg in a cast). So this confirms that osteoarthritis is much less 'wear and tear' and more 'wear and inadequate repair' to some extent.

I asked Professor Vincent about treatment hopes for the future and we'll talk more about this in a later chapter, but, in essence, we either have nothing or joint replacement surgery. Pain relief is practically all we have that sits in between these two extremes, apart from some therapies.

The best treatment is probably prevention, though. The most important things we can do to prevent osteoarthritis and ease pain are to avoid becoming overweight, keep strong and reasonably active. These are key to keeping arthritis at bay. Some experiments have shown that off-loading a knee in a certain way can help cartilage regrow. Perhaps future arthritis treatment will involve making the best of our own ability to heal or making that healing process more effective.

Let us recap a little. Osteoarthritis develops in joints where cartilage damage and changes in the mechanical properties of the joints occur, often as a result of injury. The cartilage tries to repair itself, remodels and, over time, becomes less robust. A cascade of biochemical processes occur within the joint, leading to inflammation. Over time, the cartilage becomes thin and eventually wears out altogether.

We know that osteoarthritis is more common the older we get. The question is, how do we know if we have osteoarthritis? Probably the most common symptom is pain. Our joints might be developing arthritis for some time, but if they're not hurting, we tend not to worry about them. We may have pain on movement, pain at rest or both. We might notice a reduced range of movement.

'I can't bend my knee very well these days'

Some people notice crunching or grinding when they move the joint. This is called crepitus, and once felt is often not forgotten. If you place your hand on a joint, such as the knee or shoulder, and feel a grinding vibration through the skin, this is crepitus. The once shiny, lubricated joint surface has probably long gone by this point.

Joint stiffness is common to many kinds of arthritis and osteoarthritis is no exception. I notice it if I'm running late in clinic or, perhaps more appropriately, when my patients complain of pain and stiffness after getting up from the chair. You might notice your joints changing shape over time. Knobbly knees, crooked fingers, bow legs or knock knees (where the knees bow out or touch in the middle) are not uncommon. Joints might give way. I'm often told, 'I just can't trust this leg any more' by people with knee or hip osteoarthritis.

Some people develop an effusion. This is fluid build-up and is usually found on the knee. We often refer to it as 'water on the knee'. This fluid is far more than water. Biochemical analysis of fluid found in knee effusions shows it is rich in many of the chemicals involved in repair and remodelling of cartilage. Perhaps fluid on the knee is an important part of the repair process in some types of knee osteoarthritis.

Some people develop muscle weakness. This is more a result of disuse than the diseased joint itself. Painful joints make us want to rest or avoid exercise. This can lead to reduced muscle bulk, especially if there has been a problem for a long time. The adage of 'use it or lose it' can readily be applied to the structures of the joints involved in osteoarthritis.

If you visit your doctor with a joint problem, what can you expect? The first thing I ask is, 'Tell me about what you're experiencing'. I'm going to use the knee as an example once again.

As GPs, we are all taught to listen to patients. In reality, we often butt in and go straight to asking leading questions. One study showed that doctors interrupt patients within about 12 seconds of them starting to talk. So my first task is to keep quiet, at least for a couple of minutes. We will ask you about your symptoms. Where is the pain? How long has it been troubling you? What makes it worse and, conversely, what eases the pain? Is it there all the time or is it worse with certain activities, such as movement or going up and down stairs? Have you ever injured your knee? What sorts of jobs or hobbies have you had?

We will then ask to examine the knee. This often starts from the minute I call the patient in. Watching how someone walks can tell us an awful lot about the potential difficulties. There might be a limp or a visible look of pain on the face of the person walking towards me. People will wince when sitting down or sit with their legs out straight. Watching a person rise from a chair to walk to the examination couch might give us a little insight into how that person lives his or her life. When looking at the affected area, we'll examine above and below it, look at the muscles for evidence of wasting, look at the joint itself for swelling, deformity, previous surgery or injury. We'll feel the knee to discover fluid or press to see if it hurts in places. We'll move the knee, checking the range of movement or feeling for crepitus – that grinding feeling mentioned earlier.

We might look for signs of inflammation. Inflammation is, in essence, the body's way of dealing with something it doesn't like. That might mean an injury or infection. We'll discuss this in more detail in Chapter 3.

On the whole, osteoarthritis can be diagnosed clinically – that is, from what people tell us and what we find on examination. That said, many people will go on to have an X-ray. This is often the case if onward referral to an orthopaedic surgeon or physiotherapist will be required. The X-ray will be interpreted by a radiologist, a doctor whose specialism is medical imaging. The radiologist will look to see if there is evidence of joint space narrowing, cyst formation and thickening at the ends of the bones beneath the cartilage, as well as extra spurs of bone (called osteophytes).

We'll go on to talk about treatment in Chapter 7, but once the diagnosis has been made, you may be offered pain relief, physiotherapy, steroid injections or even joint replacement surgery.

3

Rheumatoid arthritis

Although under the same umbrella, rheumatoid arthritis is quite different from osteoarthritis. You might have heard of rheumatism before. It's a word I tend not to use much these days. It is used to refer to a whole host of conditions relating to the joints and I often hear patients refer to joint pain as rheumatism or a 'touch of the rheumatics'.

Rheum is an old-fashioned word. According to the *Oxford English Dictionary* it comes from the Greek *rheuma*, meaning 'stream'. It actually refers to watery secretions of the eye and nose. In seventeenth-century France, rheumatism referred to snuffling, an outward sign of problems with the inner flow of watery humours. In essence, water flowing to the wrong places in the body.

It is understandable that early physicians might have thought this. Creaking, fluid-filled joints, hot, red and swollen – it is clear that this is due to an excess of fluid, surely? Perhaps not. While in time I'm sure people will look back at what we do with horror, I'm glad we have advanced somewhat since those olden times.

So just what is rheumatoid arthritis? Rheumatoid arthritis is an inflammatory type of arthritis. It occurs when our immune systems recognize our joints as foreign. Normally, inflammation is the way our bodies defend themselves. I often tell people that it is the way the body deals with things that could be harmful. Inflammation is an essential part of our immune response. It is a far from straightforward set of processes, occurring in the context of injury and illness. It is a protective process, responding to a vast array of potentially harmful stimuli and permits removal of these harmful stimuli and subsequent healing. It could be seen as our first line of defence against threats to our ongoing well-being.

We are probably all familiar with some of the signs of inflammation. These have been recognized since ancient times. They are known as calor, rubor, dolor, tumor, and functio laesa. To put these

17

in more familiar terms, these are heat, redness, pain, swelling and loss of function.

When I used to get tonsillitis all the time as a child, I would be all too aware of all of these features. When we injure ourselves, this is another time when we might witness this cluster of physical signs of inflammation.

Inflammation occurs in living tissue. It is the result of a complex interaction at a variety of levels in the body. From cell level, to tissue to organ system. Features such as swelling, redness and heat are brought about by a change in blood flow. The blood vessels in the affected area dilate. That is, they get wider, allowing more blood to enter the area of injury. Blood is full of good stuff to help us heal, so it is perhaps not a surprise that we need more going to the affected area. The blood vessels become leakier. Far from being a solid tube, our blood vessels allow fluid to move out of them into the surrounding tissues. This fluid contains the constituents of the immune system needed to fight whatever noxious stimulus it encounters and begin the healing process. The problem with inflammation, as many of us will contest, is that it can cause us harm. The best of intentions, but not always the best outcome.

Inflammation comes from the Latin, *inflammare*, meaning 'to set on fire'. Our own cells, blood vessels and a vast array of cellular signalling mechanisms combine to eliminate the cause of insult or injury. Dead cells and tissues are removed. Repair is initiated. However, inflammation can cause harm to otherwise healthy surrounding tissues. Inappropriate inflammation is found in auto-immune conditions, of which rheumatoid arthritis is one of many. The inflammatory process has to be tightly regulated, and for the most part it is. It is when things go wrong that normal, protective mechanisms become abnormal, and cause disease.

There are two ways to look at inflammation. We can use time-scales to differentiate them. Acute inflammation is fast, occurring within minutes to hours of the initial insult or injury. It is led by a type of immune cell called a neutrophil. Neutrophils circulate in our bloodstream and are involved in the response to injury and infection. Acute inflammation may be mild, and self-limiting if on a local level. It may produce local features, such as redness and swelling, or more marked systemic features, such as fever.

Chronic inflammation is inflammation that stays for a while, some-times lifelong. When people I meet refer to something as chronic, they often mean severe, yet the term refers to the timescale. It derives from the Greek *khronos*, meaning 'time'. Chronic inflammation is a much slower process than the acute form. It involves other cells of the immune system (macrophages, monocytes and lymphocytes) and can cause severe, progressive damage to tissues. It is often less obvious in terms of signs and symptoms, at least in the early days.

Acute inflammation is the initial short, sharp shock to the offending organism or injury. Like a flash flood or someone playing a trick on you. It's the 'boo' response from the immune system. Chronic inflammation is longer and more drawn out, like the gradually rising tide or the anxiety we might feel when something is worrying us. It is slow, drawn out, insidious.

This is perhaps why acute inflammatory responses are more obvious and why diseases such as rheumatoid arthritis may go unnoticed for some time. Chronic inflammation is a much more gradual process than the acute variety.

Acute inflammation can be triggered by a whole array of noxious stimuli. These could be bacteria, viruses, fungi, parasites, injuries or toxins. There are a number of potential outcomes from acute inflammation. These might be resolution and healing, progression (things just get worse) or death of the cells and tissues (called necrosis).

Chronic, or long-term, inflammation often has a variety of causes. It might be caused by viral infections, infection you've had for a long time (chronic infections), repeated or persistent injury, or autoimmune disease (of which rheumatoid arthritis is an example).

We mentioned earlier that chronic means long term rather than severe, but chronic inflammation can lead to severe symptoms, particularly if tissues or organ systems become damaged. Chronic inflammation could be caused by persistent injury or infection, such as an ulcer or tuberculosis. It could be due to prolonged exposure to a toxic agent or, as is the case with rheumatoid arthritis, an autoimmune disease. This can lead to tissue damage and persistent inflammation.

Rheumatoid arthritis is a chronic inflammatory condition. (I think I've mentioned this so often, it is pretty apparent by now.) It mainly affects the small joints of the hands and feet, but can occur in any synovial joint. We've mentioned these joints before. These are the joints lined with lubricating membranes. It is the synovium, the tissue that produces synovial fluid, and other parts of the joint that are affected by rheumatoid arthritis.

Rheumatoid arthritis is progressive – that is, it gets worse over time, particularly if left untreated. You might notice that people have rheumatoid arthritis, particularly those who have had the condition a long time. Take a look at the hands. There is often significant damage to the hands over time, particularly if untreated or undertreated. I'd say take a look at their feet too, but that would require some explaining.

The effects of the inflammation aren't just confined to the hands and other synovial joints. There is an increased risk of heart disease, weakened bones, anaemia and infection. Rheumatoid arthritis is the most common type of inflammatory arthritis. According to Arthritis Research UK, around 1 per cent of people in the UK have rheumatoid arthritis, and it is the second most common cause of arthritis. I suspect many of us, if not all, know someone with rheumatoid arthritis. Rheumatoid arthritis tends to become more common the older we get. Women tend to develop rheumatoid arthritis between their forties and seventies, and men from their mid-sixties onwards. Women are more likely to get rheumatoid arthritis than men.

The vast majority of people get joint pain, swelling and occasional flares of the disease. About a fifth of people with rheumatoid arthritis get a very mild form, but around 5 per cent of people develop severe disease or disability.

For the average GP, looking after around 2,000 people, we might see a new case of rheumatoid arthritis every couple of years. It might not sound like much, but it soon adds up.

Rheumatoid arthritis causes inflammation of the synovial membranes in the small joints of the hands. This is called synovitis. As we've mentioned earlier, -itis means inflammation. So the synovium becomes inflamed. Swollen. Painful. People with rheumatoid arthritis often describe stiffness, particularly in the mornings. Inflammatory pain is often worse after a period of rest and eases off after about half an hour of being up and about in the morning.

The synovium often becomes thickened and swollen. Immune cells flock to the area and new blood vessels grow. Cartilage, the shiny, shock-absorbing tissue at the ends of our bones, gets broken down. The space within the joint becomes filled with fluid. Chemical messages go awry and the joint is broken down. As to why this happens, this question has been, and continues to be, the subject of much research. There may be a genetic cause, and certain genetic links have been uncovered. We know that smokers seem to have a greater risk of developing the disease, and get more severe disease once it takes hold. So stop smoking. It isn't just your lungs that suffer (but you knew that anyway, right?)

Some relate a potential preceding infection to the development of rheumatoid arthritis. There have been some suggestions that a bacterium found in gum disease, called *Porphyromonas gingivalis* has been linked to the development of rheumatoid arthritis. That's right. Gum disease. It is thought that this organism produces a by-product that causes a process called citrullination. Certain proteins and peptides become 'citrullinated', which is a normal biochemical process in some tissues. In rheumatoid arthritis, an autoantibody forms against citrullinated proteins, causing an immune response to develop. One test we carry out to detect rheumatoid arthritis is to look for antibodies to these citrullinated peptides and proteins.

Put a little more simply, a normal part of our body undergoes a normal process. For some reason, antibodies are generated that recognize something normal as abnormal, then go on the attack. A case of mistaken identity at a microscopic level.

There are other conditions that can cause the synovial membrane to swell, not just forms of arthritis, so it isn't always quite this straight-forward. If I see someone with suspected rheumatoid arthritis, my job is to get him or her seen by a specialist as quickly as possible. If your doctor thinks you might have rheumatoid arthritis, you should ideally see a rheumatologist within a couple of weeks or so. Swelling of the small joints of the hands and feet, with more than one joint affected, with morning stiffness and perhaps pain on squeezing the knuckles together (the metacarpalphalangeal joints) gets you a trip to your local rheumatologist. Rheumatologists are specialist doctors trained in the diagnosis and treatment of joint conditions. They also deal with many rare conditions, particularly autoimmune condi-tions. At medical school we used to joke that rheumatologists deal with the bits of medicine no one else understands.

If I see someone with possible rheumatoid arthritis, what are the options for treatment? Initially pain relief: non-steroidal anti-inflammatories (NSAIDs), paracetamol or codeine, pending specialist opinion. Once formally diagnosed and seen by a spe-cialist, you might be offered steroids, to improve the symptoms, and then a type of drug called a disease-modifying anti-rheumatic drug (DMARD). We'll talk more about the different treatment options for arthritis in Chapter 7. You'll be offered physiotherapy to improve function, and occupational therapy input to improve your abilities in and around the home.

I mentioned earlier that rheumatoid arthritis doesn't just affect the joints. It can affect blood vessels, the coatings of the lungs, the sac in which the heart sits, the eyes, nerves and other parts of the immune system. Problems such as carpal tunnel syndrome, neck problems causing nerve pain, rupture of tendons (they join muscles to bone), heart disease and stroke. There's an increased risk of depression and anxiety in people with rheumatoid arthritis. Treatments such as steroids can cause the bones to become brittle. Some people get problems with their food pipe due to side effects from anti-inflammatory medications. People with rheumatoid arthritis may feel unwell much of the time. They may be tired, lose weight or have night sweats. The problem is, there are a large number of conditions with very similar symptoms.

Other conditions may cause synovitis, the inflammation of the membrane lining the joints. These include bacterial or viral infections, 'reactive arthritis' in response to infections such as sexually transmitted infections, types of gout, assorted medical problems, some of which are rather rare. This list is by no means exhaustive.

I've already mentioned what sorts of symptoms make me suspect rheumatoid arthritis. Once seen and referred for urgent assessment, we might arrange some tests. It's good for the rheumatologist to have as much information as possible on which to base a diagnosis. You'll almost certainly have a blood test. (Despite all the progress made in modern medicine, bloodletting still has a role.) We'll be looking for anaemia, evidence of inflammation, certain special tests to see if parts of the immune system are targeting your own cells (autoantibodies). We might arrange a chest X-ray or X-rays of the joints of the hands or feet. The specialist may arrange ultrasound scans or magnetic resonance imaging scans. Ultrasound scans are the kind we use for pregnant women. These scans use sound to bounce off the structures in the body and form a picture. Magnetic resonance imaging scans use super-strong magnetic fields to generate images and are really good at looking at soft tissue.

In short, rheumatoid arthritis is a common, long-term, inflammatory condition affecting our joints and a whole host of other parts of us. Recognition and prompt referral are key, and treatments are available. We'll find out more about that in Chapter 7.

4

Other types of arthritis

The most common types of arthritis I see are undoubtedly osteo-arthritis and rheumatoid arthritis. According to the Arthritis Foundation, a US organization providing information and support to people with arthritis, there are over 100 possible causes of arthritis. Some are conditions that primarily affect the joints. Others, such as rheumatoid arthritis and ankylosing spondylitis, have effects elsewhere in the body. Conditions such as Behçet's disease, degenerative disc disease, Ehlers–Danlos syndrome, myositis and pseudogout may all involve the joints.

You'll be pleased to know that I won't go into too much detail about the rare types, but I will talk about some of the more common ones we see. This chapter is about some of the less common, but important, causes of arthritis.

Ankylosing spondylitis

Ankylosing spondylitis is an inflammatory type of arthritis. It tends to affect the spine. Inflammation affects the joints and the ligaments (the structures joining bone to bone) causing pain and stiffness. This tends to be worse around the low back and buttocks. It can also affect the upper spine and the chest. Over time it can cause the joints of the back (called the vertebrae) to stick together. As we've already learnt, the spine needs to provide a point of anchor for all the structures that allow us to move, along with flex-ibility and durability. As the disease progresses, the back becomes stiffer, more rigid. This causes the spine to become inflexible.

The cause is thought, in part, to be genetic. While many of us may carry genes for a whole host of potential diseases, it is not until something is triggered that the disease develops. In the case of ankylosing spondylitis, this is a gene involved in the immune system called HLA-B27. Some experts think there might be an infec-tious cause, possibly a bacterial infection.

Many diseases, particularly those with a genetic element, work a little like a lock and a key. We can imagine the gene to be a lock. Some environmental factor, such as an infection, is the key. No lock, means no disease. No key, no disease. Combine the two, and disease develops. Over time we are beginning to understand more about the role our genes, and the environment, play in the development of disease. A case of nature *and* nurture coming into play.

We mentioned earlier that many chronic inflammatory diseases take a time to diagnose. Ankylosing spondylitis is no exception. For some, it could be years till a diagnosis is made. The symptoms may start gradually. Vague low back pain and stiffness may occur. I see back pain every day. Do I always think it might be ankylosing spondylitis? I can honestly say that it rarely crosses my mind.

The pain and stiffness tend to be worse after a period of rest. So typically, after a prolonged period of sitting, or in the morning after a night in bed. It tends to wear off after a while of being up and about. Given that this inflammatory back pain tends to be worse after rest, it's not uncommon for people to complain of pain in the early hours of the morning.

As the condition progresses, the stiffness and pain affects not just the lower back, but the upper back too, as well as the rib cage and neck. The joints that attach the base of the spine to the rest of the pelvis, the sacroiliac joints, also fuse. The end result is someone with limited flexibility and a stiff, rigid back. The rib cage begins to fuse, which may make it difficult to breathe deeply. Over time, inflammation affects the other joints. Hips, shoulders, knees, ankles, and even fingers and toes. The upshot is reduced mobility, a stooped posture, and general stiffness of many joints.

Ankylosing spondylitis tends to be much rarer than osteoarthritis and rheumatoid arthritis. It is three times more common in men than women, and tends to be found in younger people. Most people diagnosed with ankylosing spondylitis are in their mid-forties or younger. It tends to run in families.

As with rheumatoid arthritis, ankylosing spondylitis can cause problems in other parts of the body. The eyes can develop iritis (which is inflammation of the iris, the coloured bit of the eye). A painful, red eye might be noticed, with the pain worse in bright light. This occurs in about a quarter of people who develop ankylosing spondylitis. In my career, I've only really seen one or two cases of ankylosing spondylitis, and in these cases iritis has occurred.

Ankylosing spondylitis tends to cause an increase in the risk of heart disease, including narrowing of the arteries and problems with heart valves. It tends to be more severe in women than in men, and is often worse in people who smoke.

Inflammation can also affect where the ligaments join to the bones. This is called enthesitis. The joints between the ribs and the breast bone can inflame. This is called costochondritis. The ends of the bones can inflame. This is called epicondylitis. There's a pattern developing here, isn't there?

As with any suspected inflammatory arthritis, diagnosis is based on the history of the condition. Symptoms, timescales, things that make it worse, things that make it better. Blood tests to look for inflammation, medical imaging to look to see if any damage has already taken place, and a referral to your local rheumatologist are the order of the day.

Non-specific low back pain

Low back pain is pretty much what it says it is. Low back pain that has been around a long time, and was even referred to in antiquity. It could be regarded as a form of arthritis, given that it causes pain and significant problems to many people. There are countless causes. It could be the joints between the vertebrae, problems with the discs, or the vertebrae themselves. It tends to be worse in different positions, such as when bending or twisting. Specific causes include fractures of the vertebrae which can occur in the context of osteoporosis (weakened bones), injuries to the joints between the vertebrae, or a prolapsed intervertebral disc (a slipped disc). If a cause isn't obvious, we often refer to it as a 'non-specific low back pain', which I can understand doesn't sound like much of a diagnosis. It sounds slightly more medical than 'you've just got an achy back', although in truth, this is probably the case.

Low back pain either comes and goes rapidly (acute bad back, lasting less than six weeks) or comes and stays (chronic back pain, lasting more than six weeks). Regardless of the cause, low back pain is very, very common. I have it, and I see several people in every clinic with it. It is estimated that a third of the British adult population suffer from low back pain at some point in their lives. Thankfully, for many of us it doesn't cause too much of a problem. Yet around a third of us with back pain will visit our GP. Is it any wonder I see it a lot?

Back pain can cause considerable problems – even pain that isn't due to a 'serious cause'. It has been said that back pain costs the UK economy over £12 billion a year, be it through direct costs to the health service, or time taken from work. Some people end up giving up work for good. I've met many a self-employed person left in financial dire straits thanks to back pain. A simple movement, such as overreaching, or a slip and a trip and any one of us could be in this situation.

While most back pain doesn't have a life-threatening cause, it can be 'quality of life' threatening. I've been lucky with mine. A job that allows me to sit most of the time, and that doesn't involve too much heavy lifting, and I am usually well enough to be able to do the things I want. Those I meet with physical jobs often suffer the most.

Back pain can come and go relatively rapidly, or stay for a long time. It can result in disability, loss of employment and with that a loss of sense of self or role in the family. Depression is not uncommon, and many I meet become reliant on medications in the long term.

For most of us with back pain, time is probably the best treatment and recovery is usually good. Some people develop 'non-specific chronic low back pain'. It can plague us recurrently, may come out of the blue, is often severe and hard to predict. That said, most cases will settle to some degree within a year. A year is a long time to be in pain. It's a long time to need pain relief, or be out of work.

Some features of back pain mean a slow, drawn-out recovery might be more likely. People with pre-existing depression may be more severely affected. Those who struggle to look after themselves tend to end up needing more help from those of us in the trade. Those of us with unsupportive workplaces, or who do heavy physical work may struggle to make a good recovery. Those of us who don't engage in some form of physical activity or have a pre-existing medical condition tend to be prone to developing long-term low back pain.

We will talk about treatment options in Chapter 7, but one thing that has changed over the years is advice about rest. I often advise people to keep 'gently pottering'. Lying flat on a floor, or on a door taken off the hinges are no longer part of medical advice. Avoid heavy lifting, twisting or bending, but try and carry on with life as much as possible. Keep moving and avoid confining yourself to bed, as tempting as it may be. It is useful to know that keeping active isn't harmful, to understand that things may take time, and not to expect everything to get better immediately; this will help us avoid developing long-term pain or disability.

Non-specific low back pain is just that – non-specific. It could have a number of causes, can be triggered non-specifically, and may be of variable severity or duration. It could be ligaments, tendons, muscles or discs, or a combination of all of them. It could be due to posture, the type of work we do, previous injuries, or other factors such as weight gain.

Gout and pseudogout

Gout and pseudogout are two of the most common causes of joint pain I see. We've probably all heard of gout before, but pseudogout? Is it gout incognito? Same gout pain, different cause? We'll answer these questions in a slightly more serious fashion later.

I see many gout cases in my clinic. Or at least something that looks like gout. The typical presentation is a hot, red, swollen big toe joint. People often describe the pain as unbearable. Like being constantly gnawed at, or stabbed in the toe. It is usually very hard to walk when an attack is happening.

Gout is caused by problems with a chemical called uric acid. Uric acid is a result of the breakdown of purines in the body. Purines are a group of chemicals that include important components of the very DNA that makes us who we are. They are found in high amounts in certain foods, and as a result, consuming them can cause the uric acid in the body to increase, which causes problems in our joints and other organs such as the kidneys.

Before I became a doctor, I used to think of gout as the sort of problem Henry VIII would suffer from. A disease of the past, caused by rich living. The sorts of foods rich in purines include seafood such as sardines or anchovies, herring, mackerel or scallops. Sadly, so does beer. Which I love. Other foods containing purines include beef, poultry, pork and vegetables such as green peas and spinach. This list is by no means exhaustive. Purines are also found in high concentrations in offal. High intake of the fruit sugar fructose can also lead to raised uric acid in the blood. So can fasting. So a rich, relatively healthy diet can cause a rise in uric acid in the body. But so can stopping eating altogether. So that crash diet I do every January probably isn't a good idea.

Some foods, such as dairy products or coffee, and vitamin C have been shown to lower uric acid levels. Which is probably why I don't suffer from gout. Perhaps I ought to have a coffee after every pint?

A diet rich in purines can result in a rise in uric acid in the blood. In certain conditions, the uric acid can develop crystals in the joints, leading to the hot, red, painful joints that I see from time to time (in other people that is, not me). Uric acid is removed from the body via the kidneys and passed out in our urine. It is a principal constituent in the faeces of birds and reptiles. In case you ever wanted to know that. That hot, red, swollen joint has similar constituents to the kind 'gifts' left on the windscreen of my car every time I park my car under a tree. Bird poo and hot red joints. Who would have thought they'd have something in common?

As we get rid of uric acid in our urine, certain medications such as diuretics (water tablets) used in the treatment of blood pressure can cause uric acid levels to rise. Some people find that gout runs in families, and there is a genetic influence in our ability to get rid of uric acid. Oestrogen, one of the main reproductive hormones in women, seems to protect women from getting gout before they go through the menopause. Some women may find that they only develop gout after the menopause.

In general, gout affects us as we get older, and is more common in men. That said, I've a few friends who developed gout in their late thirties (see Darren's story, below). Joint infections are one of the possible causes of hot, red, swollen joints, and if we think someone has an infected joint we usually admit them to hospital. In Darren's case, thankfully, infection wasn't the case, but it took several days to work out the cause of his swollen knee and it turned out to be gout.

The diagnosis of likely gout is a clinical one. By this I mean it is diagnosed on what you say, and what we see. I may carry out tests after the gout has settled, including checking a uric acid level. I might arrange an X-ray of the affected joint to see if it could be another type of arthritis. The gold standard of diagnosis is a joint aspirate, but we tend not to carry these out in a general practice setting. In a joint aspirate, a small needle is inserted into the joint space and some fluid is removed. This is synovial fluid, and it is sent to the laboratory to look for evidence of uric acid crystals. In reality, this usually gets done in hospital by the orthopaedic or rheumatology specialists if an infection is suspected. The reason being is that any needle inserted into a joint could potentially introduce infection into the joint. Any penetration of the skin can drive normal skin bacteria into the joint. These bacteria are quite harmless when living on the skin, but could cause infection when inserted into the joint. We are a veritable ecosystem of bacteria, but they are best placed where they are supposed to be.

Some people go on to develop a condition called tophaceous gout. Having gout for a long time, or with high uric acid levels, can lead to the development of gouty tophi. Bumpy, hard growths within the joint, which are often painful. In some rare cases, with very, very high uric acid levels, kidneys can become damaged by the sheer quantity of uric acid crystals they are having to filter.

Pseudogout is caused by a different crystal. Said to be slightly less painful, but to many as equally unpleasant as gout, it is caused by the deposition of calcium pyrophosphate in and around the joint. Also producing hot, red and swollen joints, it occurs in many of the major load-bearing joints. This includes the feet, but also knees, toes, shoulders, ankles and hands. Just as gout frequently occurs in other joints apart from the big toe, so can pseudogout. It tends to happen more frequently in older people.

In the clinic, we might find it hard to tell the difference between acute gout and acute pseudogout. Either way, in the short term treatment is similar. More on that later.

Darren

Darren is a friend of mine, and we've known each other for a few years. One day, I had a message from his wife, Jo. She was worried about him, so I popped over for a chat and a cuppa. I'd been at work all day, and was pretty frazzled. As GPs, we're not allowed to treat friends or family, except in emergencies, but I didn't think there would be much wrong with popping by for a chat.

Darren had been feeling unwell. A bit of a sore throat, a fever, and his left knee had been really painful. It was swollen and warm, and red. And he'd struggled to walk on it that day at work. When I popped round, we had a bit of a chat, then I checked him over. He had an intensely swollen left knee, which was hot, warm and red. He had a fever of nearly 39 degrees Centigrade. I was worried he might have a septic arthritis, and took him to hospital.

After several hours in A&E, he was seen by the orthopaedic team and taken to a ward, so I headed back home to get some sleep before another busy day on-call. Darren stayed in hospital for five days, and was eventually diagnosed with gout.

'I stayed in the hospital,' he told me. 'They took some fluid from my knee, which showed gout crystals. They also took me to theatre for an operation. They tidied a few bits up in there from my years of martial arts.

'It still causes me problems from time to time. Whenever I get a sore throat, it tends to get sore. I saw my GP who did a blood test and started me on allopurinol. It wasn't quite enough so he increased the dose. When it flares up, I take prednisolone . . . the colchicine doesn't seem to do it for me. I know when it will cause me problems. It tends to flare up if I eat tuna, but I've started taking cherry tablets which seem to help'.

I thank Darren for sharing his story. Darren tells me that he's found taking cherry supplements very helpful in reducing the number of flare-ups he has. There is indeed a growing body of evidence to say that drinking cherry juice seems to reduce the number of exacerbations of gout. As is often the case, more research is needed, but it might provide a cheap and effective option for some.

Bursitis

Bursitis is another cause of joint pain and swelling. Bursae are sacs that cushion the movement of muscles and tendons around bony sites at the joints. A little bit like those things you put under furniture legs to slide them across floors. You know the ones. Sometimes these bursae can swell up, and I often see them when they are very large.

You might have heard of some causes of bursitis: student's elbow and housemaid's knee. Student's elbow is olecranon bursitis. Although I've never seen it in a student. The bursa overlying the olecranon – the pointy bit of the elbow – becomes inflamed, often as a result of injury – 'I clobbered my arm the other day and now it's all swollen'.

Something akin to a large egg in size, they often look rather alarming. Over time they may settle on their own. If we think it might be infected, we may take a sample of the fluid to send to the laboratory for analysis. On the whole, most settle down with nothing more than time and pain relief.

Other examples include housemaid's knee, also known as prepatellar bursitis. This occurs over the knee, and like student's elbow, I've never seen this in a housemaid. In fact, I don't think I've ever met a housemaid. This isn't the nineteenth century after all. I've seen it most commonly in plumbers and electricians. It is probably related to spending time on their knees.

The bursa in front of the kneecap becomes swollen and a little painful. It might be warm and red. Some become infected and will require a sample of fluid as taken above, as well as antibiotics. Most settle, in time, with pain relief and trying to avoid kneeling on the affected knee for a period of time. Some people may have the fluid removed and a steroid injection into the sac to prevent it from coming back, but I try and avoid this as most will get better slowly over time.

So in essence, bursitis usually settles in time, with a bit of pain relief, time, and trying to avoid the problems that cause it in the first place. Easier said than done, I know.

Degenerative disc disease

Degenerative disc disease is a term given to the general wear and tear of part of the spine that many of us suffer from as we age. In-between the vertebrae are the intervertebral discs. I liken them to stale jam doughnuts (hear me out). Discs have a soft centre with a firm outer ring and sit between your vertebrae, providing cushioning and flexibility. Over time they may wear, becoming dehydrated and narrowing. This means the vertebrae become closer together, which might lead to a nerve being pinched. This might mean the joints between the vertebrae rub together. The discs could disintegrate, or part of the soft middle could squeeze out through the tough outer casing. All of these can contribute to wear of the disc, which in some people can cause pain.

Fibromyalgia

Fibromyalgia isn't strictly an arthritis. There is no inflammation of the joints. Yet it is painful, and often presents in a similar way to many joint conditions. In the past it was regarded as a non-diagnosis. A label to give people who ached in places, who were depressed and anxious. Although still seen by some as a controversial diagnosis, we now realize it to be a definable clinical entity. Medicine likes to prove things. It likes to see it, cut it out, put it under a microscope. So we didn't believe it was a problem. Fibromyalgia doesn't show up on a scan, or make itself known on a blood test. But it is a real condition. Rather than a problem with the joints, it is a problem with the processing of pain signals in the brain.

Features of fibromyalgia include widespread pain and tenderness in the joints. People often describe full body pain. Other symptoms include problems with mood, such as depression or anxiety. There may be overwhelming fatigue. Bowel problems such as irritable bowel syndrome are common.

There have been a number of potential causes considered, but deep down, we don't really know what causes the condition. At least many of us as doctors acknowledge it to be a problem.

There are a number of factors at play. There may be a genetic predisposition. Certain neurotransmitters such as serotonin may be lacking in some places, or in excess in others. An excess of amplifying neurotransmitters and a lack of those that suppress pain may occur.

We will talk a little more about the nature of pain in later chapters. Rather than a problem with the joint, fibromyalgia is a problem with signalling and perception of pain. When I describe this, the first question I get asked is, 'Is this in my head?' The answer is . . . yes, a bit, sort of. But before I'm accused of dismissing this condition as psychological, hear me out. All human experience is 'in our heads'. From the sound of bird song, the taste of lemons, the smell of our favourite perfume or appreciation of the colour orange, all these sensations are in our heads. They are interpreted and put into context by the workings of our brains. I often tell people that we will have different memories of a consultation. Different perceptions of what is said. No one really remembers much of what I say in a consultation. They largely only remember if I've been nice to them (there's a valuable lesson in here somewhere). Without our brain to interpret sensory information, there would be no feeling. No understanding. No memory. No experience.

So everything is, in part, in our heads. Cancer, diabetes, heart disease and arthritis. They may start off in a distant part of our bodies, but they are felt with our brains. While the cause of fibromyalgia is largely unknown, special studies using brain imaging show different levels of activity in different parts of the brain of people with fibromyalgia compared to those without. Pain is felt to a similar degree, but those with fibromyalgia perceived pain to be greater in usually non-painful stimuli, with greater parts of the brain appearing active.

In terms of tests, many people may be given a diagnosis of fibromyalgia as a diagnosis of exclusion. Other causes of joint pain may have been ruled out. Scans will have shown nothing obvious, and blood tests are normal. That said, if the diagnosis is clear, we may not need many tests at all. There are a number of tender spots that are looked for to help support the diagnosis. These are either side of the neck, just where it meets the base of the skull. Around the shoulders, elbows, upper and lower back, chest, neck or abdomen. This list is by no means conclusive. We'd look for other symptoms such as fatigue and lethargy, problems with unrefreshing sleep, or problems with memory or concentration.

There's a big overlap with other conditions such as irritable bowel syndrome and depression. For some of us, it might simply be that our lifestyles cause us to be achy, have poor quality sleep or find it hard to concentrate. This is where the challenges of diagnosis arise, and possibly where some of the scepticism towards fibromyalgia as a diagnosis once developed. Treatment is available, and we'll discuss this more in Chapter 7.

Infectious (septic) arthritis

Infectious arthritis is inflammation of the joints caused by an infectious organism, usually bacterial or viral. As with many of the causes of arthritis discussed so far, infectious arthritis is either acute with a rapid onset, or chronic, staying around for some time.

In the course of my career, I haven't seen a huge number of cases of infectious arthritis. It happens, but is not anywhere near as common as osteoarthritis.

Acute infectious arthritis is a rapidly developing condition, usually affecting a single joint (but sometimes more), and affecting the synovial and surrounding tissues. In younger people, we see infectious arthritis caused by *Neisseria gonorrhoea*. That's right – gonorrhoea. It's not strictly isolated to younger people, but as gonorrhoea is sexually transmitted, older people are at a lower risk. Make of that what you will. There are many other potential causes, and it often varies between different age groups.

Young children may get joint infections caused by common skin or soft tissue bacteria such as *Staphylococcus aureus* or strepto-cocci. Viral causes, such as Parvo B16 (which causes slapped cheek syndrome), Varicella (chicken pox), HIV or Epstein–Barr virus (glan-dular fever) can occur at any age.

Bites are not an uncommon potential cause of infectious arthritis. Dog and cat bites can be fairly unpleasant, with a whole host of potential bacterial causes. Human bites can be equally unpleasant. I'm not sure what I'd be rather be bitten by, a household pet or a fellow human being? It's a close call in terms of bacterial unpleasantness.

People with underlying joint problems such as rheumatoid arthritis may be at a greater risk of developing infectious arthritis, as are those who are immunosuppressed for some reason or another. This may include people with diabetes, HIV, or on drugs that may suppress the immune system.

We might notice a rapidly swollen, painful, hot and sometimes red joint. We might notice a reduced range of movement. We may otherwise feel well, but some may notice a fever.

Gonococcal arthritis can also be linked to skin inflammation (dermatitis), multiple joint pains and inflammation of the tendons and their sheaths (the structures joining muscle to bone).

The cause is usually determined by taking a sample of synovial fluid from the joint. This is called a joint aspirate. X-rays, MRI or ultrasound scans may be organized, as might blood tests. Prompt access to treatment if very important, particularly for bacterial causes of infectious arthritis. This is because joint destruction can rapidly follow. Cartilage can be destroyed, leading to irreversible destruction of the joint.

Chronic infectious arthritis tends to be less common, and may last weeks or months. Some people are more at risk than others, such as those with rheumatoid arthritis, HIV or those on immuno-suppressant medications. Recipients of replacement joints may also be at risk of developing chronic infectious arthritis.

Chronic infectious arthritis may be less noticeable, at least in the early stages. Swelling may be mild and gradual, the joint may be only slightly warm, there may be minimal or no redness, and pain limited to a nagging ache. While the onset may be less dramatic, joint damage may still occur, with damage to the cartilage and underlying bone.

Psoriatic arthritis

Psoriatic arthritis is another type of inflammatory arthritis. As the name suggests, this occurs in people who suffer from psoriasis. Psoriasis is a relatively common skin condition. It is a chronic condition, namely that many people suffer from it for a long time.

It may wax and wane, but is treatable in a proportion of patients. It is often seen as a silvery scaly plaque overlying a red, inflamed base, usually found on the extensor aspects of the body. Namely elbows and knees. It can also occur all over the body, as well as in 'droplets', known as guttate psoriasis. The latter may occur after an infection such as a bacterial throat infection.

About a fifth of people who suffer from psoriasis may develop psoriatic arthritis. This can have a significant negative impact on the quality of life of those with the condition. People with psoriatic arthritis will often experience joint swelling and pain, much akin to other causes of inflammatory arthritis. They may go on to develop joint deformity, which for some can cause marked disability. You might recall the playwright Dennis Potter, of *The Singing Detective* fame. His main protagonist suffered from severe psoriasis. Potter himself suffered from severe psoriatic arthropathy.

As with many of the different types of arthritis mentioned thus far, it can appear in a variety of different joints. Some find the small joints, such as the hands, are affected. Some find multiple larger joints are affected. Some get arthritis in a few joints, and some only on one side of the body. Some find the disease affects the spine. The disease tends to wax and wane, with a variable pattern over time. Sometimes good, sometimes bad.

Who do we tend to see with psoriatic arthritis? I've met people at different ages and stages of life develop the condition, but in general we see people under the age of 40, with a slow, gradual onset. It might be back pain, or pain in other joints, which tends to ease off after a period of exercise or once they're up and about. A lot like the other types of inflammatory arthritis we've discussed before. There's a bit of a pattern forming here.

As with all of the causes of inflammatory arthritis we've discussed so far, early diagnosis and treatment are key. This is to minimize the severity of destruction affecting the joint. As with other causes of inflammatory arthritis, a number of other conditions are also associated with psoriatic arthritis. These include high blood pressure (hypertension), heart disease, inflammatory bowel disease, diabetes and even depression. That's not to say that people with psoriatic arthritis are destined for all of these conditions, but more that there appears to be an increased risk.

Who gets psoriatic arthritis? Having psoriasis is probably a good (or bad) place to start. The exact cause, though, is uncertain, but we see an increased risk of developing the disease in people who smoke, drink too much alcohol or are obese.

Time and time again, despite all the research that goes into diet and lifestyle, good health comes down to a good diet, avoiding becoming significantly overweight, and avoiding smoking. It might sound a little repetitive to some, but I spend most of my days in clinic emphasizing the importance of these factors.

Reactive arthritis

For most, if not all of my time, reactive arthritis was often called Reiter's syndrome. Medicine is full of eponymous syndromes and names, which, when studying, used to drive me to distraction. Anatomical names, biochemical pathways and diseases named after the great and the good, after the giants of science and discovery upon whose shoulders we stand. Something like that.

Reiter's syndrome was so named after Hans Reiter. Dr Reiter was a physician in Nazi Germany, who is said to have carried out medical experiments on the unfortunate souls held captive at Buchenwald. We should never forget the horrors of the Holocaust, but those that perpetrated horror, even if in the name of science, should perhaps not be immortalized. Not even in the pages of a medical textbook. So reactive arthritis it is.

Like the other types of arthritis so far discussed, reactive arthritis is an inflammatory process. While the trigger may be an infection, this infection is usually at a distant site, or may even have resolved to some degree. There is an increasing body of evidence to suggest that the infectious micro-organism can be found closely associated with the joints.

The usual causes are either a sexually transmitted infection or gastrointestinal cause, such as food poisoning. Potential culprits include chlamydia, the sexually transmitted infection, and gonorrhoea, as well as salmonella, campylobacter and shigella, to name but a few. The latter three cause gastrointestinal disease.

Reactive arthritis refers to a constellation of symptoms such as inflammation at the end of the water pipe (urethritis) or neck of the womb (cervicitis), joint pain and swelling (arthritis) and eye irritation (conjunctivitis). There might also be skin pustules, ulceration of the mouth, inflammation of the head of the penis and a discharge or even involvement of the heart or brain.

In the course of my career I've only met one or two people who have had a firm diagnosis of reactive arthritis, at least through a sexually transmitted cause. It does make me wonder if there are more people out there with it, but because we are seeing them later on in life, we don't think to ask about their sex lives.

Why should an infection in one place lead to swelling of joints in a distant part of the body? The mechanism is relatively poorly understood. It could be that the infectious organisms are present in the joint, making this a form of infectious arthritis, of sorts.

Why is it that some people who catch chlamydia get reactive arthritis, and some don't? You might recall earlier we talked about ankylosing spondylitis, an inflammatory condition affecting the spine. It is linked to carrying a gene for HLA-B27, which is involved in part of the immune system. This is the same gene implicated in the development of reactive arthritis. Carriers of the gene appear to have an increased susceptibility to developing reactive arthritis.

What should we look out for in reactive arthritis? Onset of stiffness and pain in a number of joints, possibly within a month or so of a new sexual partner, with a recent episode of penile discharge. In women, it is a little less obvious, for . . . well . . . obvious reasons. We can also expect to see joint pain and stiffness affecting the ankles, feet or knees. The heels are another common site of pain, and low back pain and stiffness can occur in the early stages. Around half of all those with a possible reactive arthritis may develop eye symptoms, usually in both eyes. Rather non-specific symptoms such as malaise and fatigue are also common. Malaise is a rather general term. It essentially refers to that feeling of 'not being quite right' that many of us get when we're unwell, but can't really put a finger on it.

As you can see, the symptoms of one arthritis are often very similar to the symptoms of another. Bits ache and swell, they might be hot or red, and you might feel unwell. Differentiating between all the different types of arthritis is often challenging. So we need to look for other clues that might point us in the direction of the correct diagnosis.

In reactive arthritis we might expect to find penile discharge or swelling and pain of the testicles, pointing to a genito–urinary cause. Women will often have an inflamed cervix, and as mentioned above, this is harder to spot. It might result in pain on sexual intercourse, or bleeding shortly afterwards. Either way it needs checking out.

Arthritis is more often than not asymmetrical. For some reason, one side of the body may be more affected than the other. The small joints of the hands or feet may be affected. There may be swelling at the sites of insertion of the tendons. These join muscle to bone, and this inflammation is called enthesitis. As with other causes of inflammatory arthritis, we may find swelling of the tendons within tendon sheaths. This is called tenosynovitis. Tendons run within a sheath that adds an element of lubrication to their movement. Inflammation of these structures can occur in a variety of different conditions, not just reactive arthritis. We might find the joints are tender. Eye conditions include iritis (inflammation of the iris) and conjunctivitis (inflammation of the conjunctiva). The iris is the structure at the front of the eye that is responsible for the opening and closing of the pupil. This can become inflamed, causing pain and redness. There may be a rash, much akin to that of psoriasis, affecting the genitals, tongue and feet. It may be in plaques or drops. Heart involvement may include episodes of very fast heart rate, enlargement of part of the heart, disease of certain heart valves, and even inflammation of the sac that sits around the heart, called pericarditis. Kidneys can be involved, causing inflammation called glomerulonephritis, and protein to be passed into the urine, called proteinuria. There may be small blood clots within the veins, called thrombophlebitis. The superficial veins, those close to the surface, can be inflamed, causing a red, raised, tender area following the path of a vein. (Thrombophlebitis is quite common in people with varicose veins, so don't be too worried that you might have a sexually transmitted infection if you get thrombophlebitis in long-standing varicose veins.)

In terms of recovery, most people go on to have a full recovery in about four to six months. Around half of all those developing the condition end up getting recurrent bouts of disease, with some developing quite aggressive arthritis. Once again, those carrying the HLA-B27 gene tend to get worse disease. About a sixth of people go on to have the disease for more than a year. Some will develop erosive damage of the small joints of the feet, leading to deformity. This may result in problems walking, contributing to the development of disability. Some people develop cataracts or visual impairment as a result.

The aim of treatment is quick recognition, mainly of the pre-cipitating sexually transmitted disease. Rapid assessment in a genitourinary clinic is the order of the day. We'll discuss treatment in Chapter 7.

Spinal stenosis

Again, not so much an arthritis as such, but a potential cause of back pain. Stenosis means narrowing, and you might be familiar with other conditions with stenosis in the name. We often use the term when referring to narrowed heart valves. In this case, the stenosis refers to a narrowed spinal canal. We learnt earlier that the spinal canal is the space in which the spinal cord runs. A flexible tunnel, in which runs the spinal cord which terminates to form the cauda equina, the 'horse's tail' or nerves that then go off to connect to the lower half of our body. Spinal stenosis is caused by a variety of factors. Gradual degeneration of the intervertebral discs, arthritis of the spine (called spondylosis), and other rheumatological conditions such as rheumatoid arthritis and ankylosing spondylitis can all contribute to narrowing of the spinal canal.

The narrowing of the canal can pinch or press on the spinal cord. This is most commonly seen in the lower part of the back, and is called lumbar spinal stenosis. This tends to present with back pain, also felt in the buttocks and legs, which tends to get worse in very typical situations. Walking, particularly downhill, running, climbing and sometimes standing, if severe. It tends to ease when people flex the neck (bend it forward) or sit down. As well as pain, people often notice numbness in the legs or feet. Their legs may not feel as strong, and when I examine them, I may notice reduced reflexes.

One test that people sometimes have is known as a nerve conduction study. This involves applying electrodes at certain points along the length of a nerve (don't worry, it's on the outside of the body). This procedure can help identify what sort of problem is affecting a nerve.

As with all medical complaints, the key is in the history of the condition. Most diagnoses are made on what I'm told, with the examination either confirming or refuting my initial theory. In terms of investigations, an MRI scan is probably the most useful test. Some people will have nerve conduction studies. MRI scans, also known as magnetic resonance imaging, use incredibly strong magnetic fields to provide images. They are great at showing up the detail in soft tissues. By that I mean the stuff that isn't bone.

Treatment may vary depending on the level of severity. More on that in Chapter 7.

You'll be pleased to know we're getting to the end of this chapter. The next set of conditions I'll lump in together.

Spondylosis and spondylolisthesis

Spondylosis is 'wear and repair' or osteoarthritis of the spine. Much like spinal stenosis, it can lead to pinching of nerves. Either side of the vertebrae are gaps through which the nerves leading off to our limbs and trunk pass. These are called foraminae. Extra bone growth, called osteophytes, often seen in osteoarthritis, can cause narrowing of the foraminae, causing compression of the nerve. This can result in pain, reduced sensation, numbness and tingling and in severe cases muscle wasting and weakness of the affected limb. It can cause a type of nerve pain called a radiculopathy, which tends to follow the path taken by the nerve that is pinched at the root.

The spinal canal may narrow at any point along its path, but most cases affect the bottom of the spine. This is called lumbar spinal stenosis. It might be as a result of arthritis in the spine, degenerative disc disease, or slippage of one vertebra on top of another (spondylolisthesis), as well as ankylosing spondylitis and rheumatoid arthritis. There's a pattern forming here, isn't there?

The symptoms are not unlike those we've so far encountered. They might include pain in the buttocks, thighs and calves. This is especially so on walking, running, climbing and standing. I'm not so sure about crawling. Safe to say, many people I meet who appear to have spinal stenosis often complain about not being able to walk very far without pain in their legs. There are treatments available as we will find out in Chapter 7.

Polymyalgia rheumatica and temporal arteritis/ giant cell arteritis

Most medical diagnoses sound like magic words. 'Polymyalgia rheumatica' and in a flash of smoke, a frog appears. Or something like that. Many medical names are a description of the problem in a mixture of Latin and Greek, and polymyalgia rheumatica is no exception.

It is an inflammatory process, and the cause is by and large unknown. It tends to occur later in life, and by that I mean 50-plus.

Aching and stiffness, particularly in the mornings, are key features. The condition particularly affects the shoulders, hips and muscles close by. It is an inflammatory condition, but it isn't overly clear why it occurs. It is more common in women than men.

The typical person I see with polymyalgia rheumatica is usually a woman in her seventies, with shoulder pain and stiffness. She may find it hard to reach above her head, or have tender, stiff shoulders and hips. There might be what we've described earlier as inflammatory pain – pain that is worse first thing in the morning and eases after a period of activity.

The shoulders are usually the main site of pain, followed by the hips. Other features may be noted, including weight loss and fatigue. The cause of PMR is unknown. Some studies suggest a potential infectious trigger, but by and large the cause remains elusive. Treatment is discussed in Chapter 7. Once treated, many will respond in a short time, but treatment may continue for up to a year, even longer in some cases.

PMR is linked to another condition called giant cell arteritis/ temporal arteritis. This is a rare disease, resulting from the inflammation of the medium and large arteries. Hence the term 'arteritis'. Inflammation of the arteries. But you know that now.

It usually presents with rapid vision loss. There might be tenderness over the temples of the scalp or pain on chewing. It may occur in people with an established diagnosis of PMR or arise out of the blue.

Other potential conditions that can occur with giant cell arteritis include a potentially fatal widening of the large blood vessel running from the heart (called an abdominal aortic aneurysm), a tearing of the aorta (aortic dissection), leaky heart valves (aortic regurgitation), nerve problems, heart disease in general, depression or even involvement of the brain or deafness. Personally, I've only ever seen someone present with blindness. I've met a few people in my time who I felt *might* have giant cell arteritis, but I can only recall a single confirmed case in my whole career to date.

Polymyalgia rheumatica, however, is rather common. At any one time I tend to have a group of patients with this condition. The vast majority respond very well to treatment. More on that in Chapter 7.

5

Prevention of arthritis

We've seen that arthritis is a term applied to a whole range of different conditions. They all have something in common. Pain, potential negative impacts on quality of life, and in some cases disability. It's probably a good idea to see what we can do to prevent arthritis.

In medicine we refer to risk factors for a disease. Some of these risk factors are beyond our control. They might include faults in our genetic make-up. We might be able to choose friends, but our parents are a little trickier to choose. Some risk factors are modifiable – things that we might have some degree of control over, such as our diet, how much exercise or how little we take, where we live, what we do for a living, hobbies.

Disease isn't all about the genes. It isn't all about what we're exposed to. Risk factors for disease work like the lock and key I mentioned in Chapter 3. Our genes play the role of the lock. The key represents the risk factors we can do something about. The things that are to some extent in our power to change. No key, no disease. No lock, no disease. Combine the two and the disease is unlocked. Something like that anyway.

We are probably all too familiar with the sorts of messages we hear about how to stay healthy. Eat five portions of fruit and veg a day. Don't get fat. Don't drink, don't smoke. Cut down on the junk food and get some exercise. It might come as no surprise that the sorts of things we can do to prevent bad health in general, can also help protect our joints.

We've talked about the main types of arthritis, at least the common ones I tend to see in my daily life as a GP. There are probably hundreds of different types, subtypes, and classes of arthritis, but if you're the one suffering from it, the name is almost less important than what we do about it. Saying that, as a doctor I find it useful to give something a name, as it can provide a guide to what I can do to help you.

In this chapter, we're going to find out about what you can do to help yourself, at least in terms of preventing arthritis.

Let's talk about osteoarthritis first. The 'wear and repair' arthritis that I see every day in clinic, and that many of us will develop over our lives. We've discovered that the development of osteoarthritis is much more complex than wearing out as we get older. Some of us remain remarkably arthritis free as we get older.

Is there a way we can prevent osteoarthritis? Possibly. It depends. Sort of. Maybe. A bit.

Sorry if that sounds vague, but in reality there is no single method we can say categorically prevents osteoarthritis. Development of osteoarthritis depends on the complex interaction of lifestyle and our own susceptibility to disease.

Perhaps the biggest contributing factor in the development of osteoarthritis, especially in the major weight bearing joints such as the hips and knees, is being overweight or obese. I'm in my late thirties, and I'm probably carrying a bit too much timber. I'm the ideal weight for someone who is seven feet tall. I know my knees take a bit of a pounding, especially when I run. Which I try and avoid, partly to spare triggering of seismic warnings across the globe. Like I say, I carry a little too much fat around the tummy. And probably a few other places according to my wife. (You know, she bought me a 'health tracker' for Christmas. You know the ones. A little wristband that tells you how inactive you've been all day, then guilt trips you into getting up and exercising. Perhaps I should take the hint. Anyway, I digress).

What is a healthy weight? We calculate that by referring to something called the body mass index (BMI). If you know your height and weight, you can work out your BMI using the following formula:

BMI (kg/m^2 = weight in kilograms divided by height in metres squared). A BMI of 20 to 25 kg/m^2 is classed as normal. Less than 20 is underweight, which brings with it a host of other problems; 25 to 30 is regarded as overweight, and anything over 30 is regarded as obese. It's not a perfect measurement by any stretch of the imagination as it doesn't really account for body composition. Most professional rugby teams could probably be classed as obese if you only use their BMIs, but I wouldn't say any of them are unfit or unhealthy in anyway. Nonetheless, it is a useful, albeit crude, measurement of weight in relation to height. We know that osteoarthritis is thought to be triggered by 'microtrauma', and is affected by the load going through a joint, so reducing that load may help reduce the risk of developing the condition. The take-home message? Lose a few pounds. When you've found the secret, let me know, won't you?

We learnt earlier that joints are more than just the bones, but other structures including muscles, tendons and ligaments go to form our joints. One potential risk factor for developing osteo-arthritis includes poor muscle strength. This makes sense when you think about it. Weak muscles can't protect the joint so well. The way we walk may change if we weaken, changing the way loads are applied through the joint. Good strength can help us maintain our independence as we age. I'm not talking about Arnold Schwarzenegger levels of strength. Functional strength, such as being able to stand from sitting, reach up, pull and push, is taken for granted. So keep the weight down and the muscles strong.

Our occupations and hobbies can play a significant role in the development of osteoarthritis. Again, probably due to stress and repeated low-level injury to joints. I don't know many people in manual occupations that don't hurt somewhere every day as they get old. Builders, plumbers, carpenters. All spend time repeatedly lifting, and I frequently meet people who have spent a lifetime in the construction industry with osteoarthritis. Knees, hips and shoulders particularly take a battering over a lifetime.

Hobbies, such as high-impact sports like running, football or rugby also make themselves known as we get older. Again, like manual, heavy jobs, sports cause slow, steady, repeated damage. I once heard that Alan Shearer, former England football player, had something in the region of 14 operations on his knees during his playing career. I've only had one operation in my entire life, and that was on my neck. That's probably a couple of operations a year for the duration of his playing career. I've met dancers with arthritic feet, runners with dodgy knees, horse riders with duff hips and swimmers with ropey shoulders.

Work gives us a sense of purpose, social interactions and a few quid in the back pocket. Sports foster teamwork, camaraderie, and are generally good from a cardiovascular health point of view, but play havoc on the joints.

Sometimes you just can't win.

There are some dietary factors that have, in part, been shown to help. The evidence is a bit limited and somewhat contradictory. Some studies have shown that vitamin C *might* help reduce cartilage loss, and that low vitamin D levels may increase the risk of developing knee osteoarthritis. Does that mean we need to go out and take supplements? Not unless you are truly deficient in these vitamins. What it probably tells us is that, as we've known all along, a healthy balanced diet is a good thing. It is good for our hearts, it is good for our minds, our sense of well-being – and our joints.

The old adage, 'you are what you eat', might seem old fashioned, but the more I learn about the amazing workings of the human body, the more I hold this to be true. I once heard a great piece of advice. 'Never eat anything your gran wouldn't recognize as food'. I think it was *the* Dr Phil Hammond. And don't eat too much of it. If that's all you remember about what makes a healthy diet, then you won't go far wrong.

In summary:

- don't get fat;
- eat a balanced diet;
- have a job that gives you a bit of exercise, but doesn't put too much load through your joints;
- have a hobby, but try not to get injured.

This is probably easier said than done.

Rheumatoid arthritis

Rheumatoid arthritis, like osteoarthritis, has a number of risk factors. Some we can modify; some are a little beyond our control. For instance, in the past it was felt that exposure to some of the early types of contraceptive pill may increase the risk of developing rheumatoid arthritis. With more modern forms of contraceptive pill this doesn't appear to be the case. As a rule, they tend to contain much less oestrogen than the original generation of 'the pill'. Hormone replacement therapy has been shown in some studies to increase the risk of developing rheumatoid arthritis, but other studies have found this to be inconclusive. Who said science was straightforward? Other factors potentially influencing oestrogen exposure include whether a person has had children, or breastfed their children. This appears to lower the risk of developing rheumatoid arthritis, whereas having a premature menopause appears to increase the risk of developing rheumatoid arthritis.

What practical steps does this suggest we can take to prevent rheumatoid arthritis? Um . . . get pregnant and breastfeed? Not much use if you're a man, and I wouldn't say this is the best method of preventing the development of rheumatoid arthritis.

The big modifiable risk factor for developing rheumatoid arthritis is smoking. Just don't smoke. The more you smoke, the greater your chances of developing the condition. The risk is particularly stronger in men who smoke. The good news is that stopping smoking means your risk of developing rheumatoid arthritis drops after stopping smoking. The bad news is that it takes 20 years for the risk to drop. That doesn't mean that there's no point stopping smoking.

Some studies have suggested that very high coffee intake appears to increase the risk. Which is disappointing, particularly for me. I drink pints of the stuff every day. How else would I get through a 16-hour day?

In terms of diet, the evidence is a bit of a mixed bag. Omega-3 oils, vitamins C and E, carotenoids, flavonoids and lycopene have been shown in some studies to help reduce the risk of rheumatoid arthritis, but in other studies this isn't necessarily the case. Once again, science comes to our aid by utterly confusing us.

Other risk factors for the development of rheumatoid arthritis include work stress and shift work, and, as mentioned in Chapter 3, gum disease. A bacterium called *Porphyromonas gingivalis* is thought to be involved in the citrullination process, which we discussed earlier. Many people with rheumatoid arthritis suffer from poor oral health. This might be due to other autoimmune conditions causing a dry mouth or problems with the jaw. Bacteria have been found in the synovial membranes of people with rheumatoid arthritis. This bacterium is rarely found in the mouths of healthy people, i.e. those without rheumatoid arthritis. It can evade the normal defence mechanisms of the mouth and cause gum disease. Gum disease is often a feature of rheumatoid arthritis at different stages throughout the disease.

Does good oral hygiene lessen your chances of developing rheumatoid arthritis? Perhaps. For many reasons, keeping your teeth and gums clean is a good idea. Want to reduce your chances of getting rheumatoid arthritis? Keeping your teeth clean and not smoking seem like good places to start.

Ankylosing spondylitis

Prevention of ankylosing spondylitis is a little more difficult. Given that there is a significant genetic role in developing the disease, this is a little difficult to change. You can't choose your parents after all. Ninety per cent of the risk of developing ankylosing spondylitis is down to having the HLA-B27 gene. As not everyone who is HLA-B27 positive will go on to develop ankylosing spondylitis, there might not even be much value in getting tested before the event.

Like the other inflammatory types of arthritis, ankylosing spondylitis can increase the risk of cardiovascular disease. Heart attacks and strokes, that sort of thing. So what can be reduced is our risk of such diseases if we have a sensible lifestyle. The stuff we hear all of the time. Not being too overweight, eating a balanced diet rich in fruit and vegetables and getting plenty of exercise. Yes, that old chestnut. The same advice we've been dishing out for as long as I can remember still holds.

Non-specific low back pain

For non-specific low back pain, degenerative disc disease, spondylosis and spondylolisthesis (basically the wear and repair causes of back pain) the opportunity for prevention is also a little limited. Given that these conditions, to some extent or another, depend on being on the planet long enough, there isn't a huge amount that is guaranteed to stop them developing. However, the same advice for general health still holds true. This is especially true in terms of keeping your weight down. Other issues may come into play. Avoiding injury and heavy lifting may help. If you're in a manual job, see if there are ways of reducing the amount of load you have to carry. This isn't always possible in many industries. Playing sport is a good way of keeping active and keeping the weight off, but once again, sports injuries may play a role in the development of painful back conditions.

Gout

Unlike low back pain, gout is eminently avoidable. Your lifestyle can play a significant impact on your chances of getting gout. As we've already mentioned, gout is caused by a build-up of uric acid crystals in the joints, which leads to pain and inflammation. Uric acid is derived from the breakdown of purines, which are found in our food. So reducing our purine intake can reduce our likelihood of gout. High purine foods include red meats and offal, oily fish and seafood as well as yeast extract (you either love it or hate it). Cutting down on these can make a difference. Alcohol and sugary drinks don't help either. Low purine foods include eggs and low-fat dairy products, bread, cereals, pasta, noodles, and fruits and certain vegetables. These won't have much of an impact on your uric acid levels. Foods with a moderate amount of purines include chicken, pork, lamb and beef (so that's the Sunday roast done for), asparagus, cauliflower, whole grains like bran and wholemeal bread, as well as duck, beans, dried peas and mushrooms. There doesn't seem like much left now, does there?

Once again I think the 'everything in moderation' advice our parents and grandparents gave us is probably a good idea. That's in *moderation*, not excess. If you're getting gout regularly, replace some of the higher purine food stuffs with lower purine foods, and see if it makes a difference.

In terms of pseudogout prevention, this is a little trickier. Pseudogout is a different crystal, calcium pyrophosphate. It tends to occur in older people and in already arthritic joints. So while it might not be so straightforward to reduce how often you get pseudogout, it might make more sense trying to prevent osteo-arthritis. That is, avoid being overweight or getting too much in the way of joint injuries.

Bursitis

Bursitis prevention very much depends on where you get it. Ischial bursitis (which is basically inflammation of your bum bone – you quite literally sit on it) can be helped by keeping your weight down. Bursitis of the knees can be prevented by using kneeling pads, particularly if your occupation involves spending much time on your knees, such as plumbers, electricians, carpet fitters and so on.

Fibromyalgia

Fibromyalgia is a trickier condition to prevent. Given that it could be regarded as a disorder of pain processing with strong overlaps between irritable bowel syndrome and chronic fatigue syndrome. Psychological distress may play a part in the development or exacerbation of the condition. Intercurrent illnesses may have a negative impact on a person's ability to cope with the symptoms of fibromyalgia. Is there anything we can do or a food we can eat that helps prevent fibromyalgia? Right now, I'm not so sure.

Septic arthritis

Septic arthritis is more a case of bad luck. Risk factors for developing it include diabetes, recent joint injury or surgery, having a joint replacement, or a skin infection overlying a joint replacement. An injury in the garden, a dog bite, a minor laceration, could potentially lead to joint infections. People like me giving joint injections need to be careful to ensure the area is thoroughly cleaned beforehand, lest we introduce infection into the joint. What can we do to prevent it? Try not go get injured perhaps? Try and be a bit less diabetic, or have a bit less rheumatoid arthritis. Probably isn't practical.

Psoriatic arthritis

The risk factors for the development of psoriatic arthritis are those for the other inflammatory forms of arthritis we've already discussed. Namely, smoking, excessive alcohol and obesity. You get the picture by now.

Reactive arthritis

Reactive arthritis, as we've mentioned earlier, can be caused by a number of different conditions. There are two main groups of conditions that can cause reactive arthritis. These are sexually transmitted infections and gastrointestinal disease.

In terms of sexually transmitted infections, perhaps the best way to avoid developing reactive arthritis is to practice safe sex. By that I mean using condoms . . . or having a headache . . . or perhaps just being tired or buying a bigger TV. Only one of those is a valid form of contraception.

In terms of gastrointestinal infections, it comes down to food hygiene. I didn't think I'd be talking about food hygiene in a book about arthritis. I'm also not the best person to advise on it. I'm a terrible cook. I only have one chopping board. I'm pretty sure I put raw meat at the top of the fridge. This is a bad thing apparently. At medical school I once forgot where I put a pint of milk. Some months later, I finally managed to track down the source of the smell to find a somewhat inflated two pint bottle of whole milk that had separated into layers. It was fascinating. But intensely stinky. During barbecue season, guests take their life into their own hands. Sausages with a carbon exoskeleton and a bleeding middle. Chicken so raw it clucks. I've got better, and no one has developed gastroenteritis just yet.

Basically, don't do what I do. Cook your food thoroughly. Let's not forget that not everyone who gets salmonella or campylobacter develops reactive arthritis. I've only seen a few cases in my career, or at least recognized it.

Spinal stenosis

Preventing spinal stenosis is a little more difficult. It is caused by narrowing of the spinal canal, which in essence is due to osteoarthritis of the spine. The general advice is to keep active, keep your weight down, consider your posture and stop smoking. Whether this will reduce your chance of developing spinal stenosis, or improve the situation once it has developed, this is a little harder to tell.

Polymyalgia rheumatica

Finally, prevention of polymyalgia is very difficult. We don't know what causes it, but we do know that it responds well to steroid medication such as prednisolone. It's tricky to prevent something if we don't really know what causes it.

In the next chapter, we will consider the sort of investigations we can expect if we have a possible cause of arthritis.

6

Investigations

While the diagnosis of some conditions requires nothing more than listening to the patient and a physical examination, for many conditions, a number of investigations are required. If you've ever been close to a doctor, we will more than likely want a sample of blood from you. In this chapter we highlight the main tests that you're likely to have.

Blood tests

First up, the full blood count (FBC). If you've ever watched a medical drama, the FBC is one of the barrage of acronyms shouted during an emergency. The FBC looks at the constituents of blood, and is useful in the investigation of pretty much every illness I think about. The FBC looks at a number of different constituents of blood, and the proportion of blood that is made up by those various components. One of them is haemoglobin; this is the red bit of blood that carries the oxygen around the body. It may go down in certain types of arthritis, particularly inflammatory arthritis or my certain medications such as those used for rheumatoid arthritis. The white cell count (WBC) is a measurement of the proportion of blood made up of white cells. White cells are part of the immune system, the army of the blood. There are number of different members of the white cell clan, including neutrophils, lymphocytes, monocytes, eosinophils and basophils. In reality, the cells I'm most interested in are neutrophils, and perhaps to a lesser extent lymphocytes. Neutrophils rise in number in response to a whole host of different causes. These include infection and injury. They 'eat' bacteria and other cellular flotsam. Lymphocytes tend to react to viral illness, monocytes may be raised in certain bacterial infections, and eosinophils tend to be raised in response to allergy or parasitic infection. We tend not to see too much of the latter in the UK however.

There are a number of other measurements that get carried out on our blood during an FBC that help give me an idea of what might be going on. Platelets, part of the scaffolding involved in blood clotting, tend to be raised in certain inflammatory processes, injuries or diseases of the bone marrow.

The FBC is a very useful test, but like many of the investigations I carry out, has to be placed in the context of the disease. It isn't much use on its own without a good story attached to it. Asides from diagnosis, the FBC is often monitored in people taking disease-modifying anti-rheumatic drugs (DMARDs), more on that later.

Slightly more specialized tests are used, particularly in the context of inflammatory arthritis. We discussed the concept of cit-rullination. Little extra bits added to proteins that then trigger off an autoimmune response. The immune system recognizing self as foreign. A test called anti-CCP looks for antibodies against citrullin-ated peptides that are involved in the development of rheumatoid arthritis. A positive test result might help make the diagnosis, but a negative one doesn't necessarily mean that rheumatoid arthritis isn't present. An earlier test, called rheumatoid factor, is also used to help determine whether someone might have rheumatoid arthritis. Like so many tests, it isn't perfect, and can be positive in other diseases such as syphilis and TB to name but two.

Another useful test is the erythrocyte sedimentation rate or ESR. It is incredibly simple. A blood sample is assessed for the time taken for the red cells to settle out. The longer the time, the higher the number and the more inflammation that's present. Slightly raised levels aren't always that useful, but very raised levels are a marker of disease. The exact disease once again depends on the story attached. We often see it raised in certain inflammatory arthritis types and polymyalgia rheumatica.

The C-reactive protein test, or CRP, is another commonly used test. It is referred to as an acute phase protein, and is raised in response to a large number of conditions, including acute inflam-mation such as injury or infection, or chronic inflammation such as inflammatory arthritis. It is also raised in people on hormone replacement therapy (HRT), the combined oral contraceptive pill (COCP), pregnancy, and the significantly obese.

We talked earlier about HLA-B27. HLA stands for human leuco-cyte antigen, which is part of the immune system and helps the body tell the difference between itself and a potentially harmful stimulus. Up to ten per cent of the UK population are thought to be positive for HLA-B27, and most people with ankylosing spondylitis are positive for it.

We also find it in inflammatory bowel disease (Crohn's disease, ulcerative colitis and so on) as well as psoriatic arthritis and reactive arthritis.

Therefore, it's a very useful test. It is usually one of the tests carried out by the rheumatology clinic. If it is positive, and there are other symptoms and signs to suggest one of these conditions, chances are the diagnosis is correct.

Other blood tests that may also be useful include blood cultures. In the case of infection, particularly septic arthritis, blood cultures may be taken to help identify the causative microbe. Blood is taken, drawn into glass bottles and sent into the laboratory. From here, the blood is incubated, and analysed for the presence of bacteria. These bacteria may well be identified and tested against an array of different potential antibiotics. That way, we can focus antibiotic therapy to the exact cause. Blood cultures tend to be requested during an inpatient stay. You have to be pretty unwell to need blood cultures, and as a GP I'm unlikely to be ordering them.

All the tests thus far mentioned are carried out on blood. There are other tests available that we carry out on blood. These might be liver and kidney function, a bone profile, to name but a few. All of them are done on blood, and your GP or rheumatologist will usually go through the results with you. Thankfully, despite the barrage of tests and investigations that can be carried out on blood samples, you don't need to give an armful.

Joint aspirate

One of the tests that I have mentioned previously is the joint aspirate – the removal of synovial fluid from a joint. I try and avoid this in the general practice setting, as there is a risk of introducing infection, causing a septic arthritis. It is also used to look for crystals in conditions such as gout and pseudogout. Samples are taken from the joint and sent to the lab. It is relatively easy, minimally painful (although it depends where you put the needle), and can be a useful investigation.

X-rays and scans

When investigating arthritis, more often than not, I tend to order an X-ray, usually of the affected part of the body, and occasionally of other areas. X-rays use a part of the electromagnetic spectrum, which includes radio waves, visible light, infrared and ultraviolet. X-rays are very useful at looking at bony anatomy. The properties of X-ray radiation are such that they pass through objects to varying degrees. The nature of the substance they are passing through alters the amount of absorption or scattering of the X-ray, with bones showing up better than soft tissues. This, at least, is the case in standard two-dimensional X-rays. I use X-rays to look for osteoarthritis particularly. They might show up signs suggestive of osteoarthritis, such as joint space narrowing, cysts developing beneath the cartilage, or extra bony spurs called osteophytes.

For the most part, X-rays are probably enough to help investigate a potential cause of arthritis. A CT scan, computed tomography, takes many two-dimensional slices, and turns them into three-dimensional images. As well as being useful in the diagnosis of a whole host of conditions, CT scans provide a way of visualizing anatomical structures in relation to one another. As a GP, I tend not to use these very often in the imaging of joints.

Magnetic resonance imaging, however, gives us much more information. MRI scans are done in those large, noisy tunnels that we are put through. Instead of using enormous amounts of radiation in the form of X-rays, MRI scanners use enormous magnetic fields. They are great at imaging soft tissues: the squidgy bits such as muscles, tendons and ligaments. The reason why they're so good at imaging soft tissues is that the enormous magnetic fields generated cause our protons to align. This isn't the stuff of science fiction. Protons are hydrogen ions, hydrogen is found in water, water is found in large amounts in soft tissues, and most of our bodies is soft and wet. The atoms that make up every molecule in our body have a spin, a little like the way the Earth rotates. They aren't inert or still. The magnetic field orientates the spin of these atoms so they all line up. When the magnetic field is turned off, they resort to their former state and give off energy. A detector picks this up and clever computer processing, that I don't understand, turns all this information into a picture, which gets assessed by a radiologist, who then sends me a report telling me what is wrong. MRI scanners are truly amazing pieces of kit, but not everyone enjoys having a scan. It's not invasive, not harmful, but can be a bit loud. You have to lie still for quite a while, and it's not suitable for everyone. The large magnetic fields have an interesting effect on metal things. They get . . . er . . . pulled on. If you get the chance, take a look at YouTube and search for 'metallic objects in an MRI scanner'. You will understand that you might not want to forget to empty your pockets before the machine is turned on. Metal fragments, pacemakers, assorted metallic implants, clips and stimulators all need highlighting before you're even recommended to have an MRI. If you have anything substantially metallic in you, chances are you probably shouldn't have an MRI scan.

The last type of imaging I'll introduce is ultrasound. This is the sort of scan that you may be familiar with, used commonly to image the developing baby during pregnancy. It is a safe, non-invasive way of giving us an idea about what might be going on in a joint. Different tissues reflect sound to differing degrees. Ultrasounds tend to be used to assess the degree of synovitis in a joint, or look for other potential causes of swelling and pain. They might be used to guide a needle during a steroid injection, particularly if it is a deep structure that is being injected. More on that later.

In summary, the sorts of tests carried out in terms of arthritis range from blood tests and forms of imaging. While no test is perfect, they all add up to form part of a jigsaw. Making a diagnosis is about pattern recognition, and tests are another way of helping make the pattern a little more apparent. Pain and stiffness that eases off makes me think of inflammatory causes of arthritis. Joint instability or locking makes me think more on the lines of osteoarthritis. Symptoms like a fever could mean septic arthritis, or in some cases gout.

Many conditions may present in similar fashions. Pain may be a feature in most, if not all forms of arthritis. Swelling is more or less universal. You can see that it is often difficult to make a diagnosis and that trying to find out what is wrong may take more than one appointment. Hopefully, this chapter will have reduced some of the mystery surrounding medical tests.

7

Treatment of arthritis

We've talked about the anatomy of the joint, some common forms of arthritis, and we've looked at how to reduce the risk of developing arthritis, where possible. We've discussed the sorts of tests available. By now, you should realize that medicine isn't mystery or magic. You might have also realized that the human body doesn't really work the way most of us think it does.

As I go through my career, fewer things surprise me. Yet most of us don't have the benefit of years of training or experience to guide us. Internet searches are one thing, but they can be a little unfiltered. When I enter a disease name into a search engine, most of the time it returns the most serious cause of a symptom, or the most severe case of a disease. We might find out about treatments that might not be available locally, or are subject to further investigation and research. Some of us might find treatments that sound too good to be true (and probably are), or based on pseudoscience and non-science (or nonsense).

As with most conditions, the treatment of arthritis depends very much on the type of arthritis we have. We've learnt about a few of the major, common types of arthritis, at least the ones I'm more likely to see as a GP.

Osteoarthritis

As osteoarthritis is a case of 'wear and try and repair', what treatments are available for it? Truth be told, there is a bit of a gap between pain relief and joint replacement. Unlike rheumatoid arthritis, there isn't such a thing as a disease-modifying drug in osteoarthritis. There is pain relief, physio, joint injections, then when you've 'had all you can stands and [you] can't stands no more', as Popeye would say, a joint replacement.

As a GP, my domain is early on in the diagnosis and treatment. Pain relief typically starts with paracetamol, but over recent years we've come to realize it probably isn't much cop, and as such isn't really recommended much these days. I say that, by which I mean modern guidelines don't really rate this much for pain relief, but many people I meet find it effective. There are better painkillers.

For a long time, the way paracetamol exerted a painkilling effect remained a bit of a mystery. It has existed in some form for over a century, and in 1955 paracetamol as we know it was developed. It was initially used to treat pain and fever in children. As a family with young children, we are never without a bottle of paracetamol suspension. In terms of its mechanism of action, this is still a little mysterious. It may affect the metabolism of certain parts of the inflammatory pathway (called cyclo-oxygenases), of which there are a number of forms. It is thought to act on this pathway in the nervous system, and thus have an effect on the interpretation of pain. It may interact with neurotransmitters in the brain, such as serotonin. It's not unusual for us to be uncertain how some medications work. This is especially the case for those drugs developed in the past.

As we learn more about paracetamol, we realize it probably isn't that good. This bears out in discussions I have with people about arthritis and pain relief.

In short, paracetamol can be used. It is somewhere to start at least, but I suspect over time this will fall out of favour. It is available practically everywhere, and as cheap as chips. I even saw it sold for 16p in my local supermarket, as well as in the pub toilets of my local (it was in a vending machine, I hasten to add). If you have a mild, occasional pain, then by all means try paracetamol. My patients have often reported that it doesn't do much. Probably worth it for a headache, and if it helps you, by all means take it.

The next set of medication commonly used in osteoarthritis is a class of drug called the non-steroidal anti-inflammatory drugs (NSAIDs). There are a number around, perhaps the most common one many people have heard of is ibuprofen. I also tend to use another drug called naproxen, and sometimes diclofenac. Just to confuse us, many medications have two names. A brand name, such as Nurofen, and a drug name – the one by which it is largely known, in this case ibuprofen. NSAIDs work on a part of the inflammatory pathway, affecting a group of chemicals called cyclo-oxygenases. A similar class of drug are the COX-2 inhibitors. COX meaning cyclo-oxygenase. They tend to end in '-coxib' and include drugs such as etoricoxib.

In general, the NSAIDs/COX-2s tend to work well for inflammatory pain, but aren't really a long-term solution. The reason being that, like many medications, they have side effects. They can be a little harsh on the kidneys, so we try and avoid them in people with pre-existing kidney conditions, or who are on medications that can also harm the kidneys. They can increase the risk of developing stomach ulcers. Long term, they can also increase the risk of developing heart disease. The NSAID that tends to have the least impact on this is naproxen, and as such you generally find that it is the drug of first choice.

For those who might need NSAIDs long term, or as a bridge to surgery, other medications are often prescribed. These are to act to ameliorate the long-term impact of remaining on these medications. Usually we co-prescribe a class of drug called a proton pump inhibitor. These drugs, including omeprazole, lansoprazole and esomeprazole, reduce the amount of acid in the stomach. This helps reduce the potential for the development of ulcers caused by taking NSAID medications. In terms of reducing the risk of developing cardiac disease, this is a little more difficult; hence, the choice of naproxen as the least potentially harmful option.

There are other ways of taking NSAIDs rather than by tablet form. NSAID gels can help osteoarthritis, and may be a way of reducing pain without the side effects. They are only really absorbed into the area to which they are applied, and so tend to be useful in those of us for whom tablet form NSAIDs may not be a good idea. Even though we might often co-prescribe with a proton pump inhibitor, we might be anxious about using oral NSAIDs in people who have had previous ulcers or bled from their stomachs. We might also avoid it in people on some form of anticoagulant (a medication that stops or reduces blood clotting).

There are many reasons why a certain medication might be unsuitable. Pre-existing medical conditions, allergies, or potential drug interactions are frequently encountered. When choosing a medication, all of these may be taken into account. This is why what might be right for one person, may not be right for another. For some, a daily dose of an NSAID, despite the potential side effects, is preferable to living in constant pain. I'm sure we can all understand that.

NSAIDs even come in suppository form, namely diclofenac. Personally, I tend not to use them in anything other than kidney stones. I've known some people to use them regularly for troublesome osteoarthritis, but for fairly obvious reasons it isn't a particularly popular route of administration. You know . . . where you have to stick 'em.

Other types of painkiller include the class of drug called opioids. These include drugs such as codeine, tramadol, meptazinol and morphine. In general terms, they act by binding to opioid receptors, reducing the amount of pain we feel. Some people describe still feeling pain, but not really being bothered by it. This seems to be the case for stronger opioids such as morphine. To some extent they mimic our naturally occurring opioids called endorphins. These are released in a variety of circumstances, including during the experience of pleasure.

Opioid drugs aren't without side effects. Perhaps the most common one encountered is constipation. They can also make you sleepy, and some people feel a little muddled and confused. Caution should be exercised if driving, and laws have been introduced on driving under the influence of medications, such as the opioid drugs. They can be rather addictive too. A little like the NSAIDs, they serve a purpose. They may well help reduce the amount of pain a person is in for the short term, but long-term risks of addiction make this class of drug unsatisfactory. That said, for short-term pain it works effectively. The difficulty, as is all too apparent, is that there is a gap between pain relief and subsequent joint surgery. The time in-between could be years, from diagnosis to the condition being severe enough to require joint replacement surgery, usually knees or hips. For some, long-term opioid or NSAID use is the only option, but this is often in the context of careful consideration of the options.

There are a number of different strengths and formulations of opioid drugs. They range from codeine, a rather weak opioid, all the way to morphine and oxycodone, which are much stronger. Codeine is often packaged together in the same tablet as paracetamol and is often called co-codamol, but other brand names exist. Drugs such as tramadol come in standard and long-acting formulations, as do morphine and oxycodone. Buprenorphine and fentanyl are opioids that come in a patch, which, when applied to the skin, provides a constant, low level of the drug at all times.

There are even injectable forms such as morphine and diamorphine (also known as heroin), which for rather obvious reasons aren't often used in the treatment of osteoarthritis (except perhaps during or after surgery for postoperative pain). The choice of drug depends on a number of factors. Some people are happy with tablets, but in those for whom swallowing might be difficult, or who might forget to take their tablets, then patches might be a better option. As a rule, the patches tend to be more expensive, so we are discouraged from providing them straight off the bat. We usually try tablets first.

While opioids are not a great option long term, for some they provide the only real solution until they are in a position to have joint surgery. In this case, the lowest effective dose for the shortest time is the order of the day. Given the tendency to develop constipation, they may well be co-prescribed with a laxative such as lactulose or senna, or possibly even both. Other laxatives are available. Given the addictive nature of opioids, coming off them can be a challenge. When stopping opioid drugs, particularly if you've been on them for a long time, it might be sensible to wean off slowly. The dose of opioid painkiller is slowly reduced in conjunction with support from a healthcare professional if needed. While I've met people come off opioids without help, it can be difficult. Opioid withdrawal is a fairly unpleasant experience. Nausea, vomiting, feeling fluey, hot and cold, diarrhoea, muscle cramps. You get the picture. I've had people describe is as 'bloody awful, Doc'. The severity of withdrawal tends to depend on the length of treatment with an opioid, and the odd codeine now and again is unlikely to lead to dependence. Regular opioid use for a few weeks may well lead to withdrawal symptoms when it is time to stop.

Another option for the short- to mid-term relief of osteoarthritis is steroid injections. Injections of steroid, such as Depo-Medrone or triamcinolone, mixed with a little local anaesthetic, can be injected into the joint. In my practice I tend to carry out knee and shoulder injections for osteoarthritis. These are perhaps the two main joints I tend to inject, given that knee and shoulder osteoarthritis are fairly common. The evidence base for steroid injections is somewhat variable, and there is still much uncertainty about why they should work. For some patients they represent a useful bridge to joint replacement. The most common side effect in my experience tends to be that they may not work, or perhaps not as well as intended. Bruising and a little bleeding may occur, and there is a small risk of infection. Steroid injections can cause a little blanching or reddening of the skin. My general advice is to rest the area for 24 hours, and monitor for infection for the next 48 hrs. People tend to notice an improvement straight away for a few hours – this is the local anaesthetic working – but the real impact may not be noticed for several weeks to come.

For those with severe disease, then joint replacement may be the only option. More on this in Chapter 10.

Rheumatoid arthritis

A key part of the treatment of rheumatoid arthritis is prompt recognition. Left untreated, rheumatoid arthritis can cause significant damage to joints, leading to disability and a reduction in quality of life. As we've found out, rheumatoid arthritis is a systemic condition. It affects the whole body, with dental conditions, increased risk of heart attack and stroke and a whole host of other issues.

Once suspected, rapid referral to the rheumatology department is key. Many areas have a rapid access clinic, where rheumatoid arthritis is diagnosed and treatment initiated. These clinics will often have nurse specialists and rheumatologists seeing patients and monitoring their progress. Once diagnosed and treatment started, you'll be invited back at regular intervals for assessment and management. There might be telephone clinics to assess severity of the condition over the phone. This is useful once a diagnosis is established.

There are a number of different assessment tools used in clinic. You may get asked something called a Health Assessment Questionnaire. There are a number of different versions available. In general, they look at your function, how well you can carry out a number of different activities of daily living. The sorts of activities that we all do without thinking, such as household chores, attending to personal hygiene or getting up from a chair unaided. Other tools used include scores of disease activity. They provide a snapshot of how severe the disease is at the time.

In the UK, the management of rheumatoid arthritis is usually carried on what is known as a shared care basis. In that, the drugs are started by the specialist, regular review in clinic either face to face or by phone, but with monitoring of the medications carried out by your GP.

The process is generally as follows. I see someone with suspect rheumatoid arthritis. I'll refer them to the rheumatologist, and arrange bloods (and sometimes X-rays) in advance. Once a medication has been started, regular bloods are needed, sometimes every two weeks or so, until a drug has been established. From here, reviews are carried out by the rheumatology team throughout the year, with more day-to-day care carried out in the community by your GP. If we notice that something is amiss or there are issues that we can't deal with in the community, then it's back to your rheumatology team. There may be other models of care where you live, such as a local GP who has a special interest in joint disease, or community-based specialist clinic. Either way, the principles are the same. Someone to diagnose and start treatment, and other professionals to keep an eye on things. Most, if not all of the DMARDs require monitoring, usually in the form of blood tests. Some may require blood tests before starting, and many need regular tests in the early stages of treatment. Over time, most settle down to needing monitoring blood tests every two to three months, but if you're on more than one DMARD (many people end up on a combination of DMARDs) then the tests may be more frequent. The following is a little information on some of the main medications used. It isn't exhaustive and is not substitute for reading through the leaflet you get with the medications. Read it. Then read it again. Then, perhaps once more for luck. Thankfully, most serious side effects are rare when medications are taken correctly.

All drugs have interactions, that is the effects of taking one drug with another. Many are known about, some may occur rarely and unexpectedly. When choosing what drug regime to commence, you and your rheumatology team will have to take these into account. Other factors to take into account when deciding what DMARD regimes to begin include pre-existing illnesses, underlying conditions, such as liver and kidney disease, whether you might be pregnant or not (probably a good idea to find out beforehand), if you're breastfeeding and what drug allergies you might have.

One more note to make on the DMARDs. Those taking it are at increased risk of infection. A pneumococcus vaccination before starting them is a good idea, as are booster injections when needed. This helps protect from a potential cause of pneumonia. This can be arranged at your local GP surgery, or even carried out by the rheumatology department but the exact detail of your local processes for arranging this will probably vary. Another note of caution. Those taking most DMARDs need to avoid live vaccines. These include measles, mumps, rubella, shingles, oral polio vaccine, typhoid, yellow fever and the BCG. The latter, formerly used for the prevention of TB, is rarely used these days in the UK due to being relatively poor at preventing TB. Most of us, depending on our age, will have had an MMR and polio vaccine. Yellow fever vaccines are usually given prior to overseas travel to endemic areas, and typhoid again is often used as pre-holiday vaccination. The shingles vaccine, also called varicella-zoster, is offered in the UK as part of a national programme. These programmes aren't aware of your individual health situation.

Disease-modifying anti-rheumatic drugs (DMARDs)

The first drug used is usually methotrexate. Methotrexate is used in a whole host of inflammatory conditions. It's been used in the treatment of rheumatoid arthritis for a good portion of the last 30 or 40 years. Methotrexate has a wide range of activities. It has anti-inflammatory properties and suppresses the immune system. It is a highly effective drug in the treatment of rheumatoid arthritis. Methotrexate interferes with the way folic acid is used in the body. Folic acid is a B-vitamin, and is involved in a whole host of important functions in the body, including DNA production and cell division. As such, we replace folic acid with a supplement. Methotrexate can be given as tablets or as injections. In the UK, we use a standard-size tablet. Because methotrexate can cause many side effects if taken incorrectly, using the same strength tablet but varying the number taken can make dose changes a little safer. Methotrexate is taken once weekly. It is incredibly important to adhere to the dosing instructions given by your rheumatology team. Many people I meet take their methotrexate on the same day of the week, with their folic acid later on in the week. Methotrexate is a valuable tool in the treatment of rheumatoid arthritis, but like so many drugs, it isn't without side effects. Taken in excess, it can be seriously harmful, if not fatal. I've heard of cases where people have accidentally taken it every day, and subsequently died. This is why it is important to stick to the instructions. It interacts with many drugs, particularly those that affect folic acid such as trimethoprim (a commonly used antibiotic for the treatment of urinary tract infections) so it is important to let people know that you are taking it. Because it suppresses the immune system, it may open people up to increased risk of infection. It can affect the production of blood cells, and therefore once started on methotrexate regular blood tests are needed. This usually settles down to every two or three months once regularly established. Sometimes you might be asked to miss a week's dose of methotrexate out, particularly if on another medication for a short period of time, or if you have an infection that isn't settling very quickly. Other common side effects include nausea, diarrhoea or vomiting, skin issues, or abnormalities on blood tests, such as liver dysfunction or anaemia.

No drug is without side effects, but methotrexate is a very valuable medication, and foundation of treatment in many inflammatory and autoimmune conditions. As such, there are many people on methotrexate and chances are you probably know someone who takes it.

Many people get on with taking methotrexate without too many difficulties, but if you feel that the side effects are too severe or are having other issues, it is important to bring that to the attention of a healthcare professional – be it your GP, rheumatologist or rheumatology nurse specialist. Many rheumatology teams have an advice line where you can call or leave messages for a member of the team to get back to you.

Other DMARDs are available. Some may be used in place of methotrexate if, for some reason or another, it doesn't suit you. These might be side effects or drug interactions. Some may be used in combination, but the choice of what drugs to combine is very much one for the rheumatology team.

Sulfasalazine is another DMARD used in the treatment of rheumatoid arthritis. It also exhibits effects on the process of inflammation, as well as having antibacterial properties. Unlike methotrexate, it is taken daily. Like methotrexate, it can have harmful effects and needs close monitoring in the form of blood tests every three months once established on treatment. Side effects are variable, and include dizziness, headache, tinnitus to name but a few. The most common are probably nausea and gastrointestinal disturbance. Pretty much every drug can cause a bit of a dicky tummy. Perhaps the most worrying are disorders of liver function and blood cell production; hence the need for regular blood tests to ensure the drug is well tolerated. As with methotrexate, most people get on fine with sulfasalazine. This list of side effects is by no means exhaustive, so as with all the medications listed it is important to read the leaflet included with the medication.

Another drug commonly used in the treatment of rheumatoid arthritis is hydroxychloroquine. How it works in rheumatoid arthritis is a little uncertain, but there are effects on parts of the immune system particularly those involved in signalling, as well as effects on a host of different enzymes. In short, we aren't really sure how it works, but it does in some people. There are many medications like this. It is reasonably effective and well tolerated, but it can uncommonly cause some significant side effects with eyesight, and as such it is important to pay attention to any changes in vision noticed while taking these medications. Prompt assessment by an ophthalmologist (eye specialist) may be necessary.

Azathioprine is another member of the DMARDs. It is used in severe rheumatoid arthritis, as well as to prevent rejection of organs after transplant, and in the treatment of other forms of autoimmune disease (disease where the immune system recognizes parts of the body as foreign). Before starting it, a special test called a TPMT test is required. TPMT stands for thiopurine methyltransferase. It is involved in the metabolism of azathioprine and those with low levels of this enzyme can't have azathioprine. They tend to be at much greater risk of side effects from the medication. Blood tests are carried out very frequently in the early stages of taking this medication, but once stable settle down to every three months.

As with all medications, side effects are possible. About a quarter of people may develop a reduced white cell count (part of the immune system) which may be grounds for stopping the drug. Gastrointestinal disturbance, once again, is common. Once again, I'd urge you to read the leaflet thoroughly and discuss any concerns with your rheumatology team.

Leflunomide is another drug that affects the inflammatory process and thus slows the progression of rheumatoid arthritis. Like the drugs thus far discussed, it also suppresses the immune system. The most common side effects include gastrointestinal disturbance, namely nausea, vomiting, diarrhoea and abdominal pain. Some people get rashes, headache or high blood pressure, mild weight loss or fatigue and lack of energy. Blood test monitoring may be very regularly initially, and may settle down to every three months once stable.

Ciclosporin is another drug sometimes used in rheumatoid arthritis. It is perhaps more commonly used to suppress the immune system in those who have had an organ transplant. It is a powerful immunosuppressant, and as such requires regular blood monitoring, both on initiation and as part of ongoing care. There are a number of side effects. As with many of the drugs so far considered, it can suppress white cell levels. It tends to raise fat levels in the blood, including cholesterol. Tremor and headache may occur, and the common gastrointestinal disturbance once again makes an appearance in the side effect list. (The more I think about it, the harder I find it to think of any drug that doesn't either bung you right up, or turn the taps on). There are plenty of other side effects, so as with all medications, read the leaflet thoroughly. Then again . . . and again . . . and again. There are some things that are very important to remember, and this is one of them. As with all immunosuppressants, there may be an increased risk of developing infection.

There are a number of other drugs that were once used in the treatment of rheumatoid arthritis. These include penicillamine, and gold. These had been used in the past, but with the advent of much better DMARDs such as those described, they've fallen out of favour. I've had patients tell me of times gone by when they would have their gold injections. But by and large, these drugs have been consigned to medical history, along with traction for back pain and the iron lung for polio. We still use leeches and maggots, however. Oh, and bloodletting. But not for rheumatoid arthritis, you'll be pleased to know.

Biologics and biosimilars

The next class of drugs used in the treatment of rheumatoid arthritis are the biologics and the biosimilars. I don't think it is too much of an exaggeration to say that the biologics have revolutionized the treatment of rheumatoid arthritis.

In an early lecture on rheumatoid arthritis, I met a number of people who came in to talk to us about their experiences. Some had been diagnosed with rheumatoid arthritis in the early days, when treatment was largely one of pain relief and sympathy. They suffered from marked joint destruction. Others had been on methotrexate, with a much less significant degree of inflammatory damage to their joints. Finally came a group of patients who had received some of the earlier biological therapies, and they remarked on how much of a positive impact these drugs had on their quality of life. These are certainly a good option for some, but they are not without their drawbacks. As with the DMARDs, these drugs are the realm of the specialist. Within the family of drugs called biological drugs are a group called TNF-alpha inhibitors. TNF, or tumour necrosis factor, is a molecule involved in the immune system in a variety of ways, including inflammation. Inhibiting TNF-alpha has been shown to be an effective way of reducing the severity of rheumatoid arthritis.

The TNF-alpha inhibitors include etanercept, infliximab, adalimumab, certolizumab pegol and golimumab. One thing of note – all people starting TNF-alpha inhibitors should be checked for latent TB before starting the medication. This is relatively easily done. Once again, let me state that this list is by no means exhaustive in terms of positive and negative effects, and is no substitute for speaking with your rheumatologist, or reading the leaflet enclosed with the drugs.

Etanercept was one of the earliest of this class of drug. It is given as a twice weekly injection and used for those who haven't responded to some of the medications previously tried. Main side effects include rash and effects on the eyes, but in rare cases can lead to lymphoma. TNF-alpha plays a role in causing programmed cell death, also known as apoptosis. This is an important bit of biological housekeeping, a way for damaged or faulty cells to be destroyed in a controlled manner. While rare, lymphoma can occur. There may also be potential for an increased risk of infection. As with many drugs, most people get on without too many side effects. One of the biggest drawbacks, at least in terms of the National Health Service, is the cost, which is over £600 an injection. In some parts of the world, where healthcare isn't provided free at the point of delivery, this could get very expensive indeed. Monitoring is usually a blood test every three to six months.

Infliximab is another TNF-alpha inhibitor and is usually given in combination with methotrexate. It is given as an infusion, which usually involves a regular visit to the hospital. It is a monoclonal antibody, and is part human, part mouse. For want of a better term, it is made by genetic engineering. Frequent side effects include an increased susceptibility to catching colds and other minor respiratory tract infections, reduced cell counts in the blood; some people develop depression, abdominal pain and nausea. It can make some skin conditions worse. Some people get a little discomfort at the time of the infusion. On the plus side, many people find it has a positive impact on their quality of life. It costs nearly £400 per vial, and infusions are needed at regular intervals. Monitoring once again involves regular blood tests.

Adalimumab is another TNF-alpha inhibitor, used in a number of inflammatory conditions including rheumatoid arthritis. It is given by injection every two weeks. It can increase the risk of infections, particularly respiratory tract, but also bowel, skin, urinary, joint and ear, in fact infections in general. Some skin cancers are more common, such as malignant melanoma, and white cell counts can be suppressed. Monitoring involves regular blood tests.

Certolizumab pegol is another member of this class of drug, and is given as a regular injection. Side effects include increased risk of infection, elevated blood pressure, nausea, rash, injection site reactions, pain and fever. Monitoring is with regular blood tests, usually every three to six months once established on treatment.

Golimumab is the final drug in our list of TNF-alpha inhibitors. It is given as an injection each month and like the other TNF-alpha inhibitors can increase the risk of developing infection and can affect the blood cells.

There are other biologic drugs that work by utilizing a different target in the development of rheumatoid arthritis. These include abatacept, anakinra, rituximab, tacrolimus and denosumab.

Abatacept affects a number of different inflammatory mediators made by T-lymphocytes, which are an important part of the immune system and help us respond to infection. It is given as an intravenous infusion, and as usual there are plenty of side effects, including gastrointestinal upset, headache, and high blood pressure. Once again it can increase the risk of developing infections, especially of the respiratory tract. Fatigue and tiredness may occur.

Anakinra is another drug that can be used in the treatment of rheumatoid arthritis. The National Institute for Health and Care Excellence (NICE) have advised that this drug is not recommended for use in the UK, consequently it is essentially unavailable on the NHS. It is given once daily under the skin, and at a cost of £734.44 a month, you can probably understand why it hasn't been given the green light in the UK, particularly when other drugs may be more effective in terms of both cost and clinical response. It might be available privately in clinics in your area. Infections can occur, as can disorders of the blood, such as low white cell count, gastro-intestinal disturbance, headaches and high blood pressure.

Rituximab is another mouse-human monoclonal antibody, and is used in the treatment of a number of different conditions, including severe rheumatoid arthritis. It is given as a pair of infusions, set two weeks apart. There is the risk of some fairly unpleasant reactions at the time of infusion, and the guidelines advise such infusions only to be given in the presence of full resuscitation equipment. Most patients receiving rituximab experience some form of reaction, and it tends to occur in the first 30 minutes to 2 hours after infusion. They can include itching, high blood pressure, acute airway arrowing (called bronchospasm) among just a few potential reactions, and even death. As a result many patients undergoing infusion are given an antihistamine, paracetamol and a steroid (hydrocortisone) prior to starting. It's pretty clear this isn't something that we tend to do in general practice, and requires the expertise of the rheumatology team to carry this out. As with all medications there are risks and benefits. The risks are severe side effects, but the benefits are the potential of improved quality of life and better disease control.

Tocilizumab and denosumab The final two drugs we will discuss are tocilizumab and denosumab. Tocilizumab is given as an infusion every few weeks, or as an injection under the skin. It can cause some fairly severe side effects. The most common it tends to cause are cold-like symptoms, headaches, raised blood pressure, and abnormal liver function tests. It can also cause raised cholesterol. In rare severe cases it can lead to severe infection, hypersensitivity reactions (in essence severe allergies) and an infection of the bowel called diverticulitis. Denosumab is used in the UK for the treatment of osteoporosis (weak bones), but can help reduced bone resorption in rheumatoid arthritis. There are two types of cell responsible for the maintenance of bone. They are osteoblasts that help build new bone, and osteoclasts that break it down. Denosumab stops the osteoclasts from doing their job, and hence the bones become less weak. Whether or not it will gain a licence in the UK for the treatment of rheumatoid arthritis, time will tell.

Cardiovascular risk with rheumatoid arthritis

One area of particular importance is the management of cardiovascular risk in people with rheumatoid arthritis. I've not spent too much time on it, but rheumatoid arthritis and other inflammatory forms of arthritis don't just affect the joints. As such, people with rheumatoid arthritis are at a higher risk of developing cardiovascular diseases such as heart disease and stroke. The mainstay of treatment is prevention. A balanced diet, keeping active, not smoking and avoiding becoming overweight are paramount. As part of your annual rheumatoid arthritis review, we should consider your cardiovascular risk (if it hasn't already been done). As such, you might be offered medication to lower your blood pressure, cholesterol lowering medications, or referred to local weight loss groups. I won't dwell on this too much, save to say that the treatment of inflammatory forms of arthritis is about more than just stopping issues with the joints.

In summary, the treatment of rheumatoid arthritis is one of prompt recognition and referral to the rheumatology team. From there, DMARDs are started to reduce the damage done to the joints. Methotrexate is the foundation medication, and other medications are used either in addition, or in place, depending on the response to the disease or other factors such as suitability to the drug. For severe symptoms, we have the biological medications. In many cases these make a dramatic difference to the disease but aren't without their side effects. It is a trade-off between the severity of the disease and the significance of the side effects. It's not an easy choice to make, and needs some careful consideration. It all depends on how severe the disease is. Drugs used in the treatment of rheumatoid arthritis take a little time to do their job. The biologics can take many weeks to take effect, sometimes even months. Nothing we have in our arsenal of medications makes everything go away overnight, however. Well, nothing I know of that is available now anyway.

Pain in rheumatoid arthritis

Pain in rheumatoid arthritis is treated in the same fashion as any other arthritis, using the medications we've discussed earlier. The exact choice depends on a number of factors, such as existing medical conditions or allergies, the same as any other condition. Physiotherapy plays a role in rheumatoid arthritis, as does exercise, and for some, surgery. Occupational therapy, the branch of healthcare involved in how we function in our lives, has a big role to play in the treatment of arthritis, particularly as we get older. Occupational therapists can help us live more independently in our homes; help us carry out the activities of daily living. They can even recommend adaptations to our homes in order for them to accommodate us as time goes by. Arthritis can be disabling, and changing the world around us can make a difference. Thresholds and steps can be adapted, grab handles installed, bathrooms made easier to use and aids have been designed to help us with our chores. Social services departments are another key part of the treatment of any potentially disabling condition. The more help we get in good time, the longer we will keep our independence. More on that in Chapter 11.

Steroids

For flare-ups of rheumatoid arthritis we can use oral or injectable steroids. These include drugs such as prednisolone (a tablet) or hydrocortisone (an injection). These particular steroids are used in a whole host of inflammatory conditions, and can make a difference much more quickly than some of the other medications we use. Long term, however, steroids can cause some significant side effects, such as thinning of the bones (osteoporosis), loss of muscles in the arms and legs, increased fat deposition in the abdomen, a filling out of the face, thinning of the skin, steroid-induced diabetes, and even suppression of the adrenal glands. The adrenal glands make our own internal steroids, and giving extra from outside the body can, in essence, turn them off. This is why it is important for people to know that you are taking steroids. When you are prescribed long-term steroids such as prednisolone, you are given something called a steroid card. It contains information for those who might attend to you if you become unwell. If you are on long-term steroids, it is important not to stop them suddenly. They need to be tapered off slowly in discussion with your doctor.

They are usually prescribed as a standard dose tablet, and the number of tablets varies. This helps us understand how much we are taking, as many medications come in different dose tablets. This can be quite confusing, so changing the number of tablets takes this confusion out. As an example, you might have to take eight doses of a 5 mg tablet, which is a dose of 40 mg a day, all taken in one go, and dropped down slowly every few days.

In order to offset some of the long-term side effects of steroids, we tend to use other medications. Much like taking long-term NSAIDs, we add in a proton pump inhibitor to protect the stomach lining. To protect the bones, we add in a drug called a bisphosphate, which might come in tablet form, or infusion form. The most common tablet form I tend to prescribe is called alendronic acid. It is taken once weekly, and because it can be a little harsh on the food pipe (the oesophagus) you have to take it sat bolt upright, half an hour before any other medications and food, with a good amount of water. It sounds like a bit of a faff to start with, but people soon get used to it, and it is probably preferable to osteoporosis. As a general rule, using DMARDs aims to reduce the reliance on steroids, and thus the potential long-term side effects.

Injectable steroids are often given for flare-ups of the disease, and are often given as an injection into the muscle (usually a buttock, if you were wondering). These are given in short bursts, perhaps a number of times a year, but the mainstay of treatment is to try and prevent this becoming problematic using DMARDs. Other localized steroid injections can be used to help with pain and swelling at a specific joint. Much like using steroid injections for osteoarthritis, but in much lower doses, steroids can be injected directly into joints. I tend to use a steroid called Depo-Medrone, but others are available. Small amounts are injected into the joint after careful cleaning, with rest for a day afterwards and monitoring for infection.

Ankylosing spondylitis

The treatment of ankylosing spondylitis has a number of key components. Exercise is a big component. As inflammatory pain is worse after resting, keeping active, stretching and freeing things up after a period of rest is important. Here, physiotherapy plays a key role in helping treat ankylosing spondylitis. Supervised exercise programmes have been shown to be helpful, and availability of these programmes may vary depending on location. It may be that your local gym might be able to help.

In terms of pain relief, NSAIDs are the foundation treatment. As with any medication, the lowest effective dose for the shortest amount of time is the aim, but with ankylosing spondylitis many people may require long-term treatment. As we've already mentioned, NSAIDs taken long term can affect the stomach lining, kidneys and heart adversely. As such, we choose the least bad option, which is naproxen, and add in a stomach acid tablet called a proton pump inhibitor. If you need the NSAIDs, then you need them.

There's no point living in pain if there is a choice, but it is important to understand the potential long-term implications of the medications we take. For severe cases, a rheumatology referral may be needed, and additional medications. These include drugs such as sulfasalazine and methotrexate, or etanercept, adalimumab, certolizumab pegol and golimumab. It depends on what part is affected as to which drug might be offered. Some are better for disease affecting the spine, some for disease affecting more distant parts. As with osteoarthritis and rheumatoid arthritis, standard pain relief such as paracetamol and codeine may be used if you find it beneficial. Surgical management might be offered for those in severe pain, with progressive deformity or X-ray evidence of structural damage. This would be carried out in a spinal surgery specialist centre.

Non-specific low back pain

Simple, non-specific low back pain is so very common, and for the most part easily treated. Acute back pain, lasting less than six weeks, with no apparent serious underlying cause, usually responds to simple analgesia. Most people with mild to moderate pain tend to self treat with over-the-counter pain relief such as paracetamol, codeine or NSAIDs. For some more severe cases, a short term muscle relaxant such as diazepam may be used. Diazepam is a member of the benzodiazepine drug class. These drugs are used as a short-term treatment for acute anxiety, muscle spasm, as a premedication before operations in people who are a little anxious, and in the past have been used for conditions such as restless legs syndrome. They are rather addictive if taken long term, and as such are only really used in the short term if absolutely needed.

In times past, people would take to their beds, which we've realized is probably the last thing we should do. Keeping active, 'gentle pottering', gradually building activity levels as the pain subsides. I generally advise people to avoid heavy lifting, and make sure they bend with their knees, until pain subsides. In fact, we should probably all bend with our knees. You know those manual handling courses you get sent on with work? I've been sent on a number. The first one told me to delegate lifting to someone else, which wasn't helpful. The other one had me picking up a pen from the floor as if it weighed a tonne. Most of us would probably lean over, grab the pen and wander off. When you're young, you can probably get away with it, but the whole bending your knees when you lift is important.

As someone who has back pain, I've taken my back for granted in the past. It even aches just sitting here writing this. I have chronic back pain. Which brings me nicely on to the management of chronic back pain (see what I've done there). Chronic back pain is pain lasting more than six weeks. There are a number of risk factors for developing it. Failure to respond to acute treatment, obesity, depression and heavy manual work are but a few of the potential risk factors. Treatment includes paracetamol, NSAIDs with the usual caveats, weak opioids such as codeine, and neuropathic agents. Drugs such as amitriptyline, gabapentin, pregabalin and duloxetine are useful in the treatment of nerve pain, but may be less useful for chronic, non-specific, low back pain. We'll talk about the nature of pain a little later, but these medications change the way the pain signal is interpreted at a neurotransmitter level. They help with that dull ache, electric shock, pins and needles, burning-like pain that we get with nerve pain. Physiotherapy is once again useful for chronic low back pain. You may have a specialist spine clinic or service locally. These may include specialist physiotherapists, pain specialists or even surgeons. In general, surgery is best avoided for chronic non-specific back pain, but may be offered if there is clear evidence of a reversible condition, such as nerve compression. Pain alone would probably not be sufficient to warrant surgery. One of the key skills of a surgeon is to know when not to operate.

Degenerative disc disease, spondylosis and spondylolisthesis

Degenerative disc disease, spondylosis (spine arthritis), and spondylolisthesis (slippage of one vertebra on top of another) are treated in a similar fashion. Spinal stenosis, the narrowing of the spinal canal, may be one of the areas where surgery is likely to be offered. Decompressing the space around the trapped nerve may help relieve the symptoms of nerve pain and tingling. Some may be offered injections of steroid/local anaesthetic in the short term, but this may not lead to long-term recovery. For those with significant slippage caused by spondylolisthesis also causing some stenosis or narrowing, decompressive surgery with fusion of the vertebrae may be offered. Surgery has a role in the treatment of back conditions, but depends very much on the exact causes. The role of surgery is to restore structure and function, so if pain originates without a clear cause in either of these areas, it may not be a valuable option. As a GP, I greatly value the opinions and skills of my spinal surgeon colleagues. They need a surgical 'target'.

The exact cause of back pain tends to get discovered after scans such as an MRI, so the treatment for back pain may be very similar in the early stages. Sciatica, a pain caused by compression of the nerve roots as they leave the spinal cord is very common, and treated in a similar fashion. It tends to cause nerve pain running down the back of the leg. To me it isn't really an 'arthritis' as such, and so I've not discussed it at too much length.

Gout and pseudogout

Gout flare-ups are usually treated with short term NSAIDs, colchicine or oral steroids such as prednisolone. If these aren't suitable for some reason, then paracetamol and codeine in a combination can be used. For those with recurrent episodes, allopurinol can be used to reduce the amount of uric acid in the blood stream, and failing that febuxostat. Allopurinol inhibits an enzyme called xanthine oxidase, which is involved in the production of uric acid. It is taken once a day and helps reduce the amount of uric acid circulating in the blood stream. As always, side effects are variable, but generally limited to rash and . . . you guessed it . . . gastrointestinal disturbance.

Febuxostat selectively targets xanthine oxidase to reduce uric acid levels. Some experience severe hypersensitivity reactions, and as such NICE have advised this drug be used as second choice after allopurinol in those who have not responded to allopurinol. Another drug, pegloticase, is available outside the UK for use in severe gout, but this has not been recommended for use in the UK by NICE.

Certain medications and medical conditions can make gout more likely. Some blood pressure drugs can cause gout, for example bendroflumethiazide (a member of a class of drugs called thiazide diuretics). Certain kidney diseases that make uric acid less able to be filtered out in the urine can also predispose to gout.

In addition to NSAIDs, a cold compress and a bit of rest can help. You know that old bag of frozen peas in the back of the freezer, you know the one. The one you've been meaning to bin when you next defrost the freezer, grab it, wrap it in a tea-towel to prevent it from causing cold burns, and pop it on the affected appendage. Similar treatment can be useful in acute pseudogout, but prevention is a little trickier than it is in gout. Different crystals are the causative agent, and as they tend to occur in already arthritic joints, treatment is largely one of pain relief.

Perhaps the best treatment of gout is prevention. Diet and lifestyle changes, including weight loss and reducing the purines in your diet make a massive difference. Stop smoking, get some exercise, go easy on the red meat, eat plenty of salad, go easy on the fruit (fructose, a fruit sugar can make it worse) and eating a healthy balanced diet all help. Lose a bit of weight. A bit of vitamin C in the diet (around 500 mg a day) might help, but it isn't a substitute for sustainable lifestyle changes.

Bursitis

The treatment of bursitis, for the most part is 'conservative'. If there's no suspicion of infection, we tend to suggest pain relief, rest, ice, compression and elevation. Pop your feet up for a couple of days, and give it some time. Olecranon bursitis, affecting the elbow, tends to settle over time. If it is getting worse, hot, red or swollen, it could be infected. Over-the-counter pain relief, rest, ice and gentle compression will help. Avoid putting pressure on the elbow. If it might be infected, a fluid sample might be drawn off and sent to the lab, and antibiotics started; this usually happens in a hospital setting.

Fibromyalgia

Fibromyalgia needs a multidisciplinary approach. By that I mean more than just me and my prescription pad. Tailored exercise programmes, cognitive behavioural therapy (a type of psychological therapy), relaxation techniques and physiotherapy have been shown to be effective. In terms of medication, simple pain relief such as that already described may be useful. Tramadol, a mild opioid, can be useful but brings with it side effects of drowsiness, constipation and, perhaps more troubling, addiction. Drugs such as amitriptyline, fluoxetine and duloxetine (types of antidepressant) may be useful, as can pregabalin and gabapentin. They may help reduce pain, increase function and reduce fatigue. Pramipexole is a drug that's used in a condition called restless legs, and has also been shown to be useful in fibromyalgia.

That said, for many, the non-drug options are perhaps the most useful. Addressing psycho-social factors that can contribute to the heightened feelings of pain may lead to long-term improvements. Working to help raise low mood, becoming actively involved in treatment, regular exercise and developing an understanding of pain and how to cope with it, can all help combat the symptoms associated with fibromyalgia.

Septic arthritis

The treatment of septic arthritis is pretty straightforward from my point of view. I send you to hospital. Eventually you'll get seen, either by an A&E doctor or an orthopaedic surgeon, and fluid will be taken off the joint and sent to the lab. Antibiotics will be started, and continued for anywhere up to ten days depending on the severity. Once the results are back from the lab, the choice of antibiotic will be honed to target the specific causative agent. The exact choice of antibiotic depends on local protocols and bacterial resistance patterns. Depending on the causative agent, you might expect to have teicoplanin, clindamycin, piperacillin/tazobactam, cefuroxime, gentamicin, ceftriaxone, ciprofloxacin, cefuroxime, sodium fusidate, or vancomycin. Safe to say, the combination and duration of these drugs varies on local guidelines.

Psoriatic arthritis

Psoriatic arthritis is a form of inflammatory arthritis, and as such, the treatment options are similar to rheumatoid arthritis. Again, a low threshold of suspicion on my part, and rapid referral to my rheumatology colleagues are the order of the day. Drugs such as adalimumab, etanercept and infliximab are used. In general, if both the skin and joints are involved, then a single drug that helps both is preferred. Methotrexate may be offered if both skin and joints are affected. For joint involvement, you might be offered leflunomide or sulfasalazine with the biologics offered if you haven't responded to treatment. Treatment of psoriatic arthritis often involve other professionals, such as a podiatrist for foot pain, dermatologist for skin disease, rheumatologists for joints, physiotherapy for mobility and strength, and occupational therapy to maintain independence.

Reactive arthritis

The treatment of reactive arthritis depends on the cause. If sexually transmitted, then a prompt visit to your local sexual health clinic is the order of the day. Gastrointestinal causes usually settle on their own as they are often a result of fairly common causes of food poisoning. We only need to treat them if people are struggling with the incessant diarrhoea or are compromised in some way. For the arthritis element, most settle in time with a little rest. You might need a bit of physiotherapy, an anti-inflammatory with stomach acid tablet, and for some a steroid injection into the affected joint. For those not responding, oral steroids such as prednisolone or an injection of hydrocortisone, sulphasalazine, methotrexate or azathioprine. The skin manifestations, which can be fairly unpleasant, may need dermatology input, and the ocular manifestations may need ophthalmological input.

Polymyalgia rheumatica

Polymyalgia rheumatica, as we've discovered, is a bit of a mystery. We don't really know what causes it, but we know that steroids such as prednisolone help the symptoms rapidly. As such, treatment of the condition is based to some extent on expert consensus. We know that long-term prednisolone treatment isn't really good for us, so getting to the lowest effective dose is the plan. In general, we start at a modest dose of prednisolone, say 15 mg, and wean off slowly. Preferably to zero, but some people remain on low dose steroids long term. I tend to drop to 12.5 mg, then 10 mg, then drop by 1 mg per month. Reviews should occur around a week after dropping the dose, as some people flare up as you drop the dose of steroid. Given the side effects of long-term steroids, I add in alendronic acid each week, vitamin D and calcium on the days not involving alendronic acid, and a proton pump inhibitor to protect the stomach lining. If symptoms flare up, I go back to the last effective dose and take longer to wean off. If I'm struggling, or there's something unusual about the presentation, then I tend to refer to our friendly neighbourhood rheumatologist. For some not responding to prednisolone, or for whom long-term steroids may cause harm, then methotrexate may be used. In giant cell arteritis/temporal arteritis, steroid doses are much higher, perhaps as high as 60 mg of prednisolone. If this is suspected, then rapid referral to hospital for assessment of vision by the ophthalmologists, then review by the physicians for consideration of a temporal artery biopsy (if needed) to confirm the diagnosis.

Some with PMR may benefit from physiotherapy to improve their mobility.

8

Complementary therapy

The difficulty with complementary therapy is that it isn't always obvious what it is. I know what I do might be regarded as mainstream medicine. That's fairly straightforward, but with exercises such as Pilates playing a role in the mainstream care of back pain, *tai chi* being taught in falls clinics, and massage for sports injuries, the lines are a little blurred. For the sake of simplicity, let's regard complementary therapy as treatments that aren't drugs or surgery. Which leaves it nicely vague and open to interpretation.

So what role does complementary therapy have? One of the difficulties with doing research in this area is it is difficult to provide the sorts of safeguards and controls that enable us to compare one treatment with another. The gold standard of healthcare knowledge is the meta-analysis, the consolidation of many studies, and the gold standard of studies is the randomized, double-blinded controlled trial. Basically, in comparing treatment X with treatment Y, this is done by neither patient nor doctor knowing what the treatment is, and by the subjects being allocated to one arm of the trial or another at random. This is quite tricky to do when someone is sticking needles into you, as in the case of acupuncture, or you're being massaged. You can't really have pretend massage. You can have sham acupuncture, but even so it is difficult to provide the safeguards needed to ensure that what we have when the results come in is the closest to the truth that we can detect. It is safe to say that there is a lot of stuff out there that just clearly doesn't work.

One of the best sources of impartial evidence on complementary therapy is something called the Cochrane Library. Groups of scholars across the globe carry out studies of studies, called meta-analyses, and use them to gather conclusions. There has been much research in complementary therapy carried out by Cochrane groups from all over the world. I'm going to super-summarize their findings.

Low back pain

Yoga might help a bit; it provides a small improvement in pain and function. Massage helps for a very short time, but has some side effects. Pilates can be useful in low back pain. There are some herbal treatments that might help reduce pain, but I would exercise caution in taking anything that hasn't been subjected to rigorous trials. *Caveat emptor.* Spinal manipulative therapy doesn't yield any meaningful difference in pain or function compared to other interventions. Behavioural therapies, of which cognitive behavioural therapy is just one, can help, but no one type of behavioural therapy is better than another. Chiropractic treatment can lead to mild reductions in pain and disability in the short to medium term (days to months) but is no better or worse than any other treatment in the long term. Some Chinese herbal medicines might help, but again, as with herbal remedies, I think it best to avoid. TENS machines (transcutaneous electrical neural stimulation) don't seem to have much evidence of benefit. Acupuncture doesn't seem to make much difference in acute back pain; there *might* be some benefit for chronic low back pain. Balneotherapy (basically, visiting a spa) is of uncertain benefit. Muscle energy techniques, a type of hands-on manual therapy, does not have sufficient evidence to be recommended. Therapeutic ultrasound might have a small effect, but the evidence is of a fairly poor quality. There is insufficient evidence for the use of arnica. Prolotherapy (injecting irritant substances into joint spaces) isn't supported by the evidence when used for low back pain.

Fibromyalgia

The Cochrane Library advises that psychological therapies for fibromyalgia may be of benefit. These include mindfulness, biofeedback, relaxation therapies or standard psychological therapy. Glucosamine might be useful in reducing pain.

Osteoarthritis

Chondroitin for osteoarthritis might be of benefit. Some herbal remedies might help, but once again, I would exercise caution when considering this route. TENS machines don't appear to help knee osteoarthritis.

Rheumatoid arthritis

Poor-quality evidence exists for acupuncture in rheumatoid arthritis. It doesn't make a difference to inflammatory marker levels, joint swelling or general health. It might reduce the use of pain relief. *Tai chi* seems to help increase lower limb mobility. Therapeutic ultrasound might help hand and grip strength, as might electrical stimulation in those with muscle wasting in their hands.

Evidence-based medicine

One of the challenges with any kind of treatment, be it complementary or more conventional, is establishing evidence of benefit. You may have noticed over time how medical treatments change. We don't give out antibiotics as often as we did. Conjunctivitis, sore throats, self-limiting respiratory tract infections, and even mild urinary tract infections will often get better on their own. Traction isn't recommended for back pain. You won't hear me recommending you taking a door off its hinges to lie on when your back goes into spasm. I won't be recommending a bread poultice for skin infections. We don't use gold injections for rheumatoid arthritis. Washing a knee out for knee arthritis has largely fallen out of favour. Why? Because of something called evidence-based medicine.

Medicine was traditionally the practice of quackery. Treatments with no scientific merit that resulted more often than not in the death of the patient: scented herbs to ward off miasma; leeches for basically everything; wet cupping in case you were too sanguine; and a belief that all illness was caused by an imbalance of the humours. As a doctor, I have a duty to keep up to date, and change my practice according to the evidence presented to me. Even in the past decade or so since I've been practising medicine, what I do has changed. We change our practices to fit the evidence. What we must not do is generate evidence to fit our views of how we understand the human body to work. Certain therapies, such as one involving diluting a substance down to a point where it is unlikely to be present, have no basis in science whatsoever, and probably work through the power of placebo. The placebo effect is certainly powerful, but shouldn't be the mainstay of treatment. The argument that a placebo doesn't cause harm should be tempered with the fact that if an effective treatment isn't used, then significant harm may result. I'm not anti-complementary therapy, but pro-science. Many medications I use are initially derived from plants, subjected to rigorous research and development, and trialled in standardized ways with safety a paramount feature.

As Neil deGrasse Tyson, the US astrophysicist, once said, 'the good thing about science is it's true, whether you believe in it or not'.

Should you use complementary therapies?

The evidence base for some complementary therapies is limited, or just doesn't exist. If you are considering a complementary therapy, do your homework. Is it based on sound scientific principles? If it can't be explained in simple scientific terms, I would exercise caution. If it relies on the existence of things that just don't exist, think again. If you don't really know what is in it, think again. If it proposes to be a miraculous cure for everything and anything, think again. If you decide upon a treatment, find out a bit more about the practitioner. Is the practitioner regulated by an appropriate body? Some therapies require no regulation or training at all. If you are advised to stop a well-established, tried-and-tested treatment to try something that promises much but delivers little, I would, once again, be sceptical. If you're considering herbal treatment, be very aware of what you are already taking; there may be interactions of which we are unaware, which could be considerably harmful. My main advice is, be careful, do your research and consider your options carefully.

9

Diet and exercise

There isn't a day that goes by without hearing about the latest fad, superfood or celebrity diet. It seems that the only qualifications needed to advise us on our diet are having been on the TV. If a celebrity chef advises on an ingredient, it sells out from the supermarkets in the blink of an eye. If someone vaguely famous is selling a piece of exercise equipment, you're guaranteed to find it selling in large numbers. Whether their advice or piece of kit is any good is less certain.

I think we probably know what a bad diet is. Living out of the local take-away is probably bad for us, unless it sells nothing but salad and oily fish. Packaged convenience foods, fast food, high-sugar snacks and fizzy drinks are not the stuff of a long and happy life. Fat probably isn't the demon we once thought it to be; sugar certainly isn't great. The moral of this story – moderation – just like your granny told you.

The question is, what is good for us if we suffer from arthritis? Whatever diet you follow, make sure you don't get too heavy. Keep your weight within healthy limits, with a BMI of less than 25 kg/m^2. If you're trying to lose weight, make sure you do it slowly and steadily. Slow, steady and small changes to your diet will be more sustainable than radical changes.

We've already mentioned that the mainstay of treatment of gout is to adopt a low purine diet. If your dinner table looks like that of Henry VIII, with rich meats and plenty of ale, you're eating the wrong food.

The challenge is, the diet that's good for gout isn't quite compatible with the diet that's good for rheumatoid arthritis.

There's a growing body of evidence that shows that fish oils are beneficial in rheumatoid arthritis. Oily fish can be high in purines, so if you've got both rheumatoid arthritis and gout then you're a bit stuck.

Fish rich in oil include sardines, mackerel, herring, fresh tuna, salmon and snapper. These are rich in the omega-3 oils that have been shown to help reduce inflammation in rheumatoid arthritis. The British Dietetic Association (BDA) recommends two portions of oily fish a week. A portion is a small fillet, or about 140 g. I'm pretty sure it doesn't count if you cover it in batter and deep fry it. Some eggs and bread advertise themselves as being rich in omega-3 oils. Borage oil, evening primrose oil and linseed oil also contain omega-3 oils. Supplements do exist, and can be sourced from high street health food stores and many supermarkets.

The much touted Mediterranean diet has been shown to have a variety of health benefits and it is also recommended for rheumatoid arthritis. This is a diet rich in oily fish, vegetables and fruit, peas, beans, nuts and seeds. According to the BDA, ensuring adequate iron intake may help with fatigue caused by low iron levels. Lean red meat in moderation; eggs (again in moderation); leafy green vegetables such as spinach; pulses; and some fortified breakfast cereals (although choose wisely as I'm not sure the garish, brightly boxed, brightly coloured sugar-coated stuff my kids crave is that good for you). As the BDA point out, vitamin C helps us absorb iron, so citrus fruits and vitamin C rich vegetables might help. Bone strength is important for all of us, so try and ensure a good calcium intake. This includes skimmed milk, green leafy veg (there's a pattern developing here), yoghurt and a little cheese, as well as nuts, sardines and pilchards. A little vitamin D, either in a supplement or with a little moderate sun exposure might help. Be wary, though, as DMARDs, the drugs taken for rheumatoid arthritis, can cause increased sensitivity to sunlight.

In terms of research, a recent study called the TOMORROW study suggests that monounsaturated fatty acids (found in olive oil, avocados and nuts) may play a role in the suppression of inflammation found in rheumatoid arthritis.

In terms of osteoarthritis, keeping a sensible weight is key in reducing symptoms. Again, the Mediterranean diet may well help with this, but more so in terms of keeping your weight down than any direct effect on the disease. There is variable research for a variety of herbal remedies, and certain foods such as green tea, turmeric, ginger and pomegranate might have anti-inflammatory properties. In terms of evidence, it's a bit dicey, so I would probably suggest a healthy balanced diet, based on the Mediterranean diet, and don't go too mad with the ginger. I mean I like it, but I wouldn't add it to everything I eat in the hope it might help with osteoarthritis. I'd be better off losing a few pounds than having a gingerbread man.

Exercise is another lifestyle intervention that helps arthritis in general. Granted, you won't want to run a marathon during a flare-up of gout, but exercise is an important part of a healthy lifestyle. It cannot be underestimated how good a bit of physical activity can be. The research talks about land-based exercise and water-based. Land-based exercise includes supervised exercise, be it individual or in groups, or self-directed exercise programmes. In general, supervised exercise seems to yield better results, but something is better than nothing.

Water-based exercise is exactly that. It might include supervised hydrotherapy with a physiotherapist, or simple swimming or aqua aerobics. It takes the load off the joints due to the buoyancy provided by the water. It might not be quite as good as land-based exercise in terms of improving cardiovascular fitness or aiding weight loss, but everything you do will help over time. The best form of exercise is the one you're doing.

Exercise, be it a walk around the block, or a visit to the gym, has beneficial effects. It's good for the heart, helps keep the weight down, gets you out and about, and helps with depression. Depression isn't uncommon in long-term illness and we know that physical exercise improves mood.

In terms of what sort of exercise, how much and when, I would suggest a pragmatic approach. Work within your limits. If it hurts too much, ease up. Start gradually, then build up. Lower-impact exercise might benefit your joints better than high-impact exercise. Walking and cycling tend to reduce the amount of strain placed on the load-bearing joints such as the hips and knees, whereas running and jogging might be better for the heart, but you'll know about it later when your knees remind you of their existence.

In terms of inflammatory arthritis, you might want to wait for a flare-up to settle before you exercise in any major way. But once settled, regular exercise will help. This is particularly the case for the other structures that make up the joints. Keeping your muscles strong, and keeping moving are key to staying well and living an independent life. The advice is, do what you can, as often as you can.

Physiotherapy is a very effective way of learning what exercises may benefit your joints. Physiotherapists can provide tailored advice and exercise to help you manage your condition. Focused regimes aimed at improving function and reducing pain can do just that. Physiotherapy availability varies depending on your location. You might have a rapid access clinic, they might be the first person you see instead of your GP, they might be the person you meet before you are seen by the orthopaedic surgeon. In terms of efficacy, mainly, it comes down to you. I prescribe tablets, and give advice. With physiotherapy, the improvement comes from you. A tablet might ease the pain for a short while, but physio may help in the long term. If you're given a list of exercises, you would be wise to do them. If you're having any difficulties with them, mention it to your physiotherapist who will be able to advise. In general terms, the sorts of exercises you will get offered are functional in nature. They use everyday movements that you need to carry out your life, and expand on them. Exercises such as standing from a seated position unaided, or squats, are valuable in keeping the thigh muscles strong. Exercises based on reaching up help strengthen the shoulders.

One well-tested exercise regime is the Otago exercise programme. Developed by Professor John Campbell and Clare Robertson at the University of Otago in Dunedin, New Zealand, this regime aims to improve strength and balance in those at risk of falls, or who have fallen. There are many potential causes of falls, and arthritis is one of them. Classes are available in many places around the UK, with supervised trained instructors. They may even be offered as part of a structured falls clinic.

10

Surgery

If other treatments aren't successful or if your arthritis is severe enough, you might be offered surgery. The type of surgery and the operation planned depend greatly on the type of arthritis and the symptoms encountered.

If we start with osteoarthritis first, perhaps the most common surgery encountered is joint replacement surgery. In 2016 alone there were more than 220,000 joint replacements in England and Wales. The most common is probably a knee replacement at around 110,000 operations a year; followed closely by hip replacement surgery at a little over 104,000 operations. Shoulder surgery is a distant third, and a few elbow and ankle replacements are carried out.

Joint replacement surgery has the ability to make a significant difference to our quality of life. When is the right time for surgery? It very much depends on how unwell you are, and how great an impact your arthritis is having on you. There are scoring systems available that help give you an idea of how severe the condition is, such as the Oxford Hip and Knee scores. Some parts of the UK require these to be of a particular severity before surgery is carried out. Other parts of the UK demand that people lose sufficient weight in order to reach a BMI cut-off point. Surgery will only be offered once you reach that cut-off. In my part of the UK, this cut-off is 35. For many, this is difficult to achieve, particularly if they have difficulty exercising, or there other reasons as to why they can't lose weight. You may be offered a supervised weight control programme, and I have known of people losing enough weight to improve their symptoms to the point where surgery can be delayed for some significant time.

Surgery might be offered if you're struggling to look after yourself, or getting severe pain, particularly at night. Once referred, your surgeon will be able to discuss with you the issues surrounding this.

Some areas may have specialized joint replacement classes prior to surgery. In these you may meet physiotherapists, nurse specialists and even previous patients who can advise you what to expect.

What happens after your referral?

Once referred, you'll have an initial appointment with a member of the team. In my area, physiotherapists carry out referrals to our orthopaedic colleagues, as a proportion of conditions may improve before surgery is even needed. When you meet the surgeon, you'll discuss your symptoms, have your X-ray reviewed and be examined. If surgery is decided upon, you'll get listed for the operation and in time brought to a pre-assessment clinic. Again, local processes may vary, but in general you'll be seen by a nurse specialist or doctor and your health issues discussed. Your regular medications will be discussed, so it's important you bring a list. You may have a blood test, an electrocardiogram (ECG), and depending on your underlying health, other tests such as a chest X-ray and an echocardiogram. An echocardiogram is a type of scan, using sound waves, that builds a picture of the structure and function of the heart. It is useful in looking at how heart valves work and how good the heart is at pumping. You may subsequently meet an anaesthetist if there is potential for anaesthetic risk. If any previously undiscovered health conditions are uncovered, you may well be sent back to your GP for further treatment. Examples include new-onset heart rhythm disturbances such as atrial fibrillation, or perhaps new high blood pressure, or under-controlled diabetes. Ideally, we should make sure your health is optimized prior to surgery, but this isn't always possible. This is especially the case if there has been some time between your consultation with your GP and your appointment in hospital. Issues such as infections will need to be cleared up before you have your operation.

Your anaesthetic options will depend on your underlying health. Some may be offered a general anaesthetic; some a spinal anaesthetic. This might particularly be the case if you have severe underlying health conditions making a general anaesthetic unwise. If you're having a spinal anaesthetic, you may be given a sedative to help you relax. I've had a number of patients tell me they've fallen asleep. Either that or spent much of their time chatting to the anaesthetist.

You'll be wheeled in, anaesthetized in whatever fashion, and wheeled out sporting a brand new piece of metal work. Recovery depends on a few technicalities: how well you are beforehand, what sort of replacement you've had, other pre-existing medical conditions and so on. But the aim is, in time, to improve your quality of life and reduce pain, and for many people I meet who have had such surgery this is entirely the case. So much so, they usually go on to have another one done. I once met someone who had five hip replacements in her time.

Hip replacements

Hip prostheses usually consist of a cup that fits into the existing hip socket, give or take a bit of chiselling; an inner plastic liner; a ball and a stem. The stem goes down the shaft of the femur (the thigh bone). Younger or more active people usually have an uncemented implant. These allow bone to grow into the implants, but recovery time may be a little longer – perhaps as long as three months. Cemented implants are usually reserved for older people. They tend to bed in fairly quickly. With life expectancies rising all the time, and obesity, it isn't unheard of for people to need revisions of previous joint prostheses.

Knee replacements

Knee joint replacement implants are equally numerous in make, but for the most part they either come in a full or half knee. For some, only part of the knee is worn, and as such only one compartment of the knee is replaced. This is often the inner (medial) compartment. There are a wide range of makes and models of replacement implant, but the most common I tend to encounter in my patients is something called a total knee replacement. The upper and lower parts of the knee joint are replaced in their entirety. An upper part slots onto a lower part covered in a plastic coating to lubricate the joint and allow movements.

Shoulder, elbow and ankle replacements

Shoulder replacements are less common, but over the course of my career I've met a few people who've had them. These implants consist of a socket that attaches to the shoulder blade and a ball and stem, much akin to a smaller hip replacement. Another option involves attaching a ball to the shoulder and having the socket on the upper arm. The exact choice of implant depends on many factors, and your surgeon will be best placed to advise on this. Elbow and ankle replacements are less common, but the principle is more or less the same – an artificial articular surface lining each side of the joint.

Other options

There are other options available. For people with osteoarthritis of the ankle, fusion is an option. This is an alternative to joint replacement and reduces pain by stopping movement at the ankle joint. Most people cope perfectly well with a slightly reduced movement at the ankle, and it is an effective means of helping ankle arthritis. In the past, cartilage surgery on the knee was popular, but over time this has fallen out of favour. I've met people with terrible arthritis who had their cartilages removed altogether in their youth. Hindsight is a wonderful thing.

After your operation

One thing you need to be aware of is what you can or can't do post-operatively. You might have a new knee, but it's different. What is normal for you will change. You might not be able to kneel down on the new prosthesis or you may need to be careful with your new hip. You'll be advised by your surgical team what might be different. It's worth knowing in advance that things will be a little different from now on.

Spinal surgery

In terms of spinal conditions, surgery is usually reserved for those with a definitive surgical target. Spinal stenosis has considerable impact on function and quality of life. There are a whole range of different operations available. Laminectomies free up space by removing a part of the vertebrae called the lamina. A discectomy may involve the removal of a little part of disc to relieve pressure on a nerve root. A spinal fusion involves the joining of one vertebrae to another. In general terms, the process is much as described above. Initial consultation, recommendation for surgery, or otherwise as is often the case, pre-assessment clinic and finally the day of surgery.

11

Keeping independent

Arthritis can be debilitating. Over time, some of us will develop an element of disability as a result of the disease. It isn't something we want to have to face, but as time goes by we all become aware that none of us is immune from the ravages of time and illness. One common difficulty I encounter is one of independence or, rather, loss of it. We start our lives needing help and support from our parents. As we age we become more independent. We spend the vast majority of the middle part of our lives personally independent. We can wash and dress, we can get out and about when we want to, we can visit friends or family, or go on holiday. Over time we may find it more difficult to carry out the tasks we previously took for granted.

Many people I meet resist getting help in good time. They resist getting help for as long as possible, until it is too late. This help can take the form of care alarms to get help in the event of falls. It might be getting carers in to help you with personal care. It could be simple things such as grab rails by the door, half-height steps or ramps. It might be walking aids or assistive technology to help you open jars, or put on your shoes.

By 2030, it is estimated that one-third of the UK's population will be over 65 years of age. We don't like to think about it, but aging does bring with it disease, or at least an increased risk of it. Being aware of this, and being prepared for a 'silver' future, can help us keep independent for as long as possible. These days there are a whole host of companies selling all manner of equipment to help keep us well and independent; from large-handled cutlery to mobility scooters and all things in-between.

Where am I going with this? Don't be afraid to ask for help. Get it sooner rather than later. Hurrying to get a care package together on a Friday night before a Bank Holiday weekend is not easy. Talk to your local social services department and get a care assessment. Social services departments can be very helpful in assessing what your care requirements might be. Get in touch with your local Citizens Advice Bureau and see if you might be eligible for benefits. They usually have a benefits adviser who can provide information on how to claim for any entitlements you might be missing out on.

There is no need to suffer. Independence is one thing, but stoicism doesn't necessarily win you any favours. There are a whole host of organizations out there, and I've included a few contact details at the end of the book.

12

Pain

As a doctor in training I was always told that 'pain is what the patient tells you it is'. We all refer to an entity we call 'pain'. A common experience but at the same time unique to each of us: we are the only person feeling that pain at that moment.

Telling someone else how we feel is complicated. It might seem simple at first thought, but it is rife with nuance and ambiguity. We feel something, such as pain. We turn it into words. 'It's a sort of aching throb in my knee. Sometimes it feels like a burning pain.'

As a doctor we listen to that description, and turn it into a pathological process. A disease, a diagnosis, and a plan of treatment. The metre or so between myself and the patient can inject misunderstanding as well as shared understanding. A feeling, buried deep within a person, relayed by nerves to the brain, turned into words, turned into a disease process and a plan of action in the brain of another person. All in a few minutes in meetings between doctors and patients across the land, millions of times a day.

Is it any surprise that sometimes we don't always understand what's going on?

Why do things hurt? What is the value of pain?

Pain is important to us. It warns us that something may be wrong. It tells us that an action or object may be harmful to us. It provides us with a survival benefit. We are built to survive, to pass on our DNA to the next generation. A sort of diluted fragment of immortality. We are the result of generations of ancestors hooking up, getting frisky, and passing their DNA down the generations. Without pain, we wouldn't know that some of the things, people, places or large bitey thing, our ancestors came into contact with could be dangerous, possibly kill them, or in some way prevent their DNA from being passed onto the next generation. Pain is useful. A bit. At the time of injury, it is very useful. Years down the line, it might tell us something is wrong, or has been wrong, but that's not very useful if we still need to get on with our lives.

We may have removed ourselves from the dangers of our ancestors, be it a millennium ago or only a few generations. We tend not to need to hunt for our food or run from potential predators. We still need to know that something might burn or sting, but we could probably do without that nagging pain in that dodgy knee, or the pain in our hands every morning, which we might suffer from with certain types of arthritis. Acute pain brings benefit. We remove ourselves from the immediate potential cause for harm. Chronic, long-term pain is a bit of a nuisance. I might know I have arthritis somewhere, but I don't want to be reminded of it when I'm tying up my shoes, or picking something up off the floor.

There are two types of nerve fibre that relay pain. One fast pain fibre, which gives us that immediate 'ouch' reaction. You know the one. I get it every Sunday when I do the ironing and accidentally brush against the iron. Every time, I tell you. This is followed by a nagging, dull pain, relayed by a slower type of nerve fibre. The pain that remains for a time after the initial insult.

How chronic, long-term pain develops is subject to much research. Nerve fibres may become activated at much lower thresholds, meaning things that shouldn't hurt cause pain. There may be areas of the brain that become active in those with long-term pain conditions that don't activate in others. There are complex interactions between emotional states, past experiences, mental health and the development of long-term pain.

Traditionally, the medical profession was fairly poor at treating chronic pain. Regardless of the cause, people with long-term pain conditions have usually been intensively investigated. We would respond with, 'There's nothing we can find wrong', only to be met with, 'Then why am I still in pain?' Medicine is much better at dealing with what it can see, rather than what other people can feel. I can tell people what isn't wrong very easily, but getting a definitive diagnosis is sometimes a bit of a challenge.

In terms of physical pain, we've discussed the medication options. Paracetamol at one end; opioids at the other. Neuropathic agents such as amitriptyline, gabapentin or pregabalin. Steroid injections to cut down inflammation, for example. For those who find these methods unsatisfactory or unsuccessful, there are pain clinics. The route into these varies, but they aim to look at pain not just in terms of the physical but also the emotional element of pain. How we feel, our mood and mental well-being can have a direct impact on our interpretation and ability to cope with pain. People with depression suffer more pain, yet people in long-term pain may be more likely to become depressed. Quite often I find the treatment of depressive illness goes hand in hand with treating pain. Pain clinics may offer injections, such as facet joint injections for spinal disease, or nerve root blocks in those with nerve root compression. What many do is offer a way of understanding long-term, chronic pain. A way of mentally and emotionally coming to terms with a form of pain that medicine doesn't quite understand as well as we'd like it to.

13

What does the future hold?

The term arthritis encompasses over a hundred different diseases and conditions. As a GP, I tend to see the forms of the condition that we've discussed in this book, yet there are countless others that I haven't covered. Childhood forms of arthritis, rarer causes of joint pain such as adult-onset Still's disease, Behçet's or intra-articular bleeds from haemophilia. It doesn't mean they're any less important, or any less debilitating. There's a fairly clichéd phrase we use in medicine when considering the likelihood of a particular diagnosis: 'Common things happen commonly'. Which is why I've discussed the more common forms of the condition.

Many of us suffer from the affliction of nostalgia. A pain for a past lost, perhaps a happier time. When it comes to the development of medical technology, the future is usually better. I don't really look back to the past and wish we treated disease like we did 40 years ago. In the future, people will look back at what we do currently with wry amusement or complete horror.

As we've discussed, osteoarthritis is treated with painkillers or surgery. There's a gap in terms of disease modification. Research groups across the world are looking at ways to identify markers of disease activity (called biomarkers) and find how to influence the development of osteoarthritis. Not everyone will get osteoarthritis, although some days in clinic it feels like everyone has it. In time we will treat osteoarthritis in a different way, perhaps developing blood tests that will allow us to diagnose it with much greater accuracy. Perhaps with drugs that will directly alter the disease process. Drugs directed to the changes that occur in the cartilage, that directly affect the function of chondrocytes, changing the way they try and remodel cartilage. Maybe we'll be 3D printing joint prostheses in the future, directly tailored to our anatomy?

In terms of rheumatoid arthritis, the biologics seem to be the area of research, and there are more currently in development. The two big issues are potential for side effects some of which are serious, and perhaps just as importantly for the NHS, the significant cost.

With an aging population, we may find technology becoming more usual in our care. Home-monitoring systems to check we are safe already exist, to some degree. Domestic robots may one day become commonplace, from simply keeping an eye on us, to providing elements of personal care. Exo-skeleton suits, powered either to permit carers to provide for us with ease, or worn by us to enable us to stand and live independently. It might be the stuff of science fiction, but these things are all in development. With this aging population will come the need for greater self-reliance and community cohesion. We will all need to help look after each other going forward.

Arthritis is a considerable cause of disease and disability, but in time this won't always be the case. The use of joint replacement surgery can dramatically improve people's lives. Simple changes to diet can have a massive impact on gout, and we're beginning to understand how diet impacts rheumatoid arthritis.

Hopefully you'll now have a greater understanding about your arthritis. You'll have an idea of how your body works, and why things go wrong. You'll have a little insight into the drugs that might be involved, as well as what you can do to prevent arthritis. Above all, I hope you can now see how what you do has a direct impact on your health.

Thank you.

Useful addresses

There is a plethora of organizations to help support you. With any diagnosis, it feels like you're the only person with it, yet, regardless of the type of arthritis you have, you'll be one of a large number. Sometimes knowing there is support out there can help you cope more easily with a long-term condition. The following are the details of a number of organizations that might be able to offer you help and support.

Social Services Department

Many councils have a dedicated phone line for their Social Services Department. One of the things that you might be able to get help with is sourcing local social care. This might be in the form of domiciliary care, such as someone who can help you with your personal hygiene, morning or bedtime routine if your conditions are getting the better of you.

Arthritis Research UK
Copeman House
St Mary's Court
St Mary's Gate
Chesterfield S41 7TD
Tel.: 0300 790 0400
Email: enquiries@
arthritisresearchuk.org
Website: www.arthritisresearchuk.
org

A charity that raises funds for research into the disease. It provides information and support for those with arthritis.

Arthritis Care
Floor 4
Linen Court
10 East Road
London N1 6AD
Tel.: 020 7380 6500 Helpline: 0808 800 4050

Email: info@arthritiscare.org.uk
Website: www.arthritiscare.org.uk

A UK-based charity supporting those with all types of arthritis.

Arthritis Action
56 Buckingham Gate
London SW1E 6AE
Tel.: 020 3781 7120 or 0800 652 3188
Email: info@arthritisaction.org.uk
(members: members@
arthritisaction.org.uk)
Website: www.arthritisaction.org.uk

A national charity that aims to provide practical support and advice for those with arthritis.

British Association of Occupational Therapists and Royal College of Occupational Therapists
106–114 Borough High Street
London SE1 1LB
Tel: 020 7357 6480
Website: www.cot.co.uk

The organization that represents occupational therapists and can provide information on finding local ocupational therapy services.

British Dietetic Association
5th Floor
Charles House
148/9 Great Charles Street
Queensway
Birmingham B3 3HT
Tel.: 0121 200 8080
Email: info@bda.uk.com
Website: www.bda.uk.com

Chartered Society of Physiotherapy
14 Bedford Row
London WC1R 4ED
Tel: 020 7306 6666
Email: Use form on website
Website: www.csp.org.uk

The organization that represents physiotherapists in the UK.

Citizens Advice
3rd Floor North
200 Aldersgate Street
London EC1A 4HD
Tel.: 03000 231 231
Website: www.citizensadvice.org.uk

There are branches throughout the UK.

National Rheumatoid Arthritis Society
Ground Floor
4 Switchback Office Park
Gardner Road
Maidenhead SL6 7RJ
Tel.: 0845 458 3969 or 01628 823524 Helpline: 0800 298 7650
Email: General: enquiries@nras.org.uk Helpline: helpline@nras.org.uk
Website: www.nras.org.uk

A charity supporting those with rheumatoid arthritis.

Psoriasis and Psoriatic Arthritis Alliance (PAPAA)
PO Box 111
St Albans
Hertfordshire, AL2 3JQ
Tel: 01923 672837
Email: info@papaa.org
Website: www.papaa.org

Supports people with psoriasis and its associated joint disease, psoriatic arthritis.

UK Gout Society Secretariat
PO Box 90
Hindhead GU27 9FW
Email: info@ukgoutsociety.org
Website: www.ukgoutsociety.org

Offers information and advice factsheets for those with gout.

Bibliography

Agca, R., Heslinga, S., Rollefstad, S., Heslinga, M., McInnes, I., et al. (2016) 'EULAR recommendations for cardiovascular disease risk management in patients with rheumatoid arthritis and other forms of inflammatory joint disorders: 2015/2016 update', *Annals of the Rheumatic Diseases*, 76(1): 17–28.

Alentorn-Geli, E. and Puig, L. (2012) 'Osteoarthritis in sports and exercise: risk factors and preventive strategies', in Rothschild B. (ed.) *Principles of Osteoarthritis – Its Definition, Character, Derivation and Modality-Related Recognition*. INTECH Open Access Publisher.

Almeida, C., Choy, E., Hewlett, S., Kirwan, J., Cramp, F., et al. (2016) 'Biologic interventions for fatigue in rheumatoid arthritis', *Cochrane Database of Systematic Reviews*.

American College of Rheumatology (2015) 'Western Ontario & McMaster Universities Osteoarthritis Index (WOMUOI)'. Available online at: <www./Western-Ontario-McMaster-Universities-Osteoarthritis-Index-WOMAC>.

American College of Rheumatology (2017) 'Reactive arthritis'. Available online at: <www.rheumatology.org/I-Am-A/Patient-Caregiver/Diseases-Conditions/Reactive-Arthritis>.

Arthritis Foundation (2016) 'Degenerative disc disease'. Available online at: <www.arthritis.org/about-arthritis/types/degenerative-disc-disease/>.

Arthritis Foundation (2017) 'Inflammatory Arthritis'. Available online at: <www.arthritis.org/about-arthritis/types/inflammatory-arthritis/>.

Arthritis Foundation (2017) 'Osteoarthritis prevention: what you can do'. Available online at: <www.arthritis.org/about-arthritis/types/osteoarthritis/articles/oa-prevention.php>.

Arthritis Foundation (2017) 'Sources of arthritis pain'. Available online at: <www.arthritis.org/living-with-arthritis/pain-management/understanding/types-of-pain.php>.

Arthritis Foundation (2017) 'Types of arthritis'. Available online at: <www.arthritis.org/about-arthritis/types/>.

Arthritis Information (2012) 'Fibromyalgia – overview and clinical manifestations'. Available online at: <www.hopkinsarthritis.org/arthritis-info/fibromyalgia/>.

Arthritis Information (2013) 'RA pathophysiology'. Available online at: <www.hopkinsarthritis.org/arthritis-info/rheumatoid-arthritis/ra-pathophysiology-2/>.

Arthritis Research UK (2017) 'Drugs'. Available online at: <www.arthritisresearchuk.org/arthritis-information/drugs.aspx?l=T#alphalist>.

Arthritis Research UK (2017) 'Polymyalgia rheumatica'. Available online at: <www.arthritisresearchuk.org/arthritis-information/conditions/polymyalgia-rheumatica.aspx>.

Arthritis Research UK (2017) 'Protease biochemistry'. Available online at: <https://oacentre.kennedy.ox.ac.uk/research/protease-biochemistry>.

Arthritis Research UK (2017) 'The inflammatory arthritis pathway'. Available online at: <www.arthritisresearchuk.org/arthritis-information/inflammatory-arthritis-pathway.aspx>.

Arthritis Research UK (2017) 'What treatments are there for ankylosing spondylitis (AS)?' Available online at: <www.arthritisresearchuk.org/arthritis-information/conditions/ankylosing-spondylitis/treatments.aspx>.

Bartels, E., Juhl, C., Christensen, R., Hagen, K., Danneskiold-Samsøe, B., et al. (2016) 'Aquatic exercise for the treatment of knee and hip osteoarthritis', *Cochrane Database of Systematic Reviews*.

Bingham, C. and Moni, M. (2013) 'Periodontal disease and rheumatoid arthritis', *Current Opinion in Rheumatology*, 25(3): 345–53.

Birrell, F., Howells, N. and Porcheret, M. (2011) 'Osteoarthritis: pathogenesis and prospects for treatment'. Available online at: <www.arthritisresearchuk.org/health-professionals-and-students/reports/topical-reviews/topical-reviews-autumn-2011.aspx>.

Bomer, N., Cornelis, F., Ramos, Y., Lakenberg, N., van der Breggen, R., et al. (2014) 'The effect of severe exercise on knee joints: identifying pathways involved in cartilage degradation processes following mechanical stress', *Osteoarthritis and Cartilage*, 22: S311–S312.

Boyden, S., Hossain, I., Wohlfahrt, A. and Lee, Y. (2016) 'Non-inflammatory causes of pain in patients with rheumatoid arthritis', *Current Rheumatology Reports*, 18(6): 30.

Brainiacstore (2008) 'BRAINIAC science abuse – John Tickle walks on custard'. Available online at: <www.youtube.com/watch?v=BN2D5y-AxIY>.

Braun, J., van den Berg, R., Baraliakos, X., Boehm, H., Burgos-Vargas, R., et al. (2011) 'Recommendations for the management of ankylosing spondylitis', *Annals of the Rheumatic Diseases*, 70: 896–904.

Breedveld, F. (2000) 'Leflunomide: mode of action in the treatment of rheumatoid arthritis', *Annals of the Rheumatic Diseases*, 59(11): 841–9.

British Pain Society, The (2016) 'An alliance of professionals advancing the understanding and management of pain for the benefit of patients'. Available online at: <www.britishpainsociety.org/>.

Brouwer, R., Huizinga, M., Duivenvoorden, T., van Raaij, T., Verhagen, A., et al. (2014) 'Osteotomy for treating knee osteoarthritis', *Cochrane Database of Systematic Reviews*.

Cameron, M. and Chrubasik, S. (2013) 'Topical herbal therapies for treating osteoarthritis', *Cochrane Database of Systematic Reviews*.

Cameron, M. and Chrubasik, S. (2014) 'Oral herbal therapies for treating osteoarthritis', *Cochrane Database of Systematic Reviews*.

Cameron, M., Gagnier, J. and Chrubasik, S. (2011) 'Herbal therapy for treating rheumatoid arthritis', *Cochrane Database of Systematic Reviews*.

Carville, S., Arendt-Nielsen, S., Bliddal, H., Blotman, F., Branco, J., et al. (2007) 'EULAR evidence-based recommendations for the management of fibromyalgia syndrome', *Annals of the Rheumatic Diseases*, 67(4): 536–41.

Cattano, N., Barbe, M., Massicotte, V., Sitler, M., Balasubramanian, E., et al. (2013) 'Joint trauma initiates knee osteoarthritis through biochemical and biomechanical processes and interactions', *OA Musculoskeletal Medicine*, 1(1): 3.

CDC (2017) 'Rheumatoid arthritis (RA)'. Available online at: <www.cdc.gov/arthritis/basics/rheumatoid.htm>.

Choy, E. (2003) 'Interleukin 6 receptor as a target for the treatment of rheumatoid arthritis', *Annals of the Rheumatic Diseases*, 62 (Suppl. II): ii68–ii69.

Choy, E. (2012) 'Understanding the dynamics: pathways involved in the pathogenesis of rheumatoid arthritis', *Rheumatology*, 51(suppl 5): v3–v11.

Chung, C. (2008) 'Managing premedications and the risk for reactions to infusional monoclonal antibody therapy', *The Oncologist*, 13(6): 725–32.

Coakley, G. (2006) 'BSR & BHPR, BOA, RCGP and BSAC guidelines for management of the hot swollen joint in adults', *Rheumatology*, 45(8): 1039–41.

Combe, B. (2016) 'SP0183 2016 Update of the EULAR recommendations for the management of early arthritis', *Annals of the Rheumatic Diseases*, 75(Suppl 2): 44–45.

Conversation, The (2017) 'The science of medical imaging: X-rays and CT scans'. Available online at: <http://theconversation.com/the-science-of-medical-imaging-x-rays-and-ct-scans-15029>.

Corbett, M., Rice, S., Madurasinghe, V., Slack, R., Fayter, D., et al. (2013) 'Acupuncture and other physical treatments for the relief of pain due to osteoarthritis of the knee: network meta-analysis', *Osteoarthritis and Cartilage*, 21(9): 1290–8.

Costa, B. da, Nüesch, E., Kasteler, R., Husni, E., Welch, V., et al. (2014) 'Oral or transdermal opioids for osteoarthritis of the knee or hip', *Cochrane Database of Systematic Reviews*.

Costa, B. da, Nüesch, E., Reichenbach, S., Jüni, P. and Rutjes, A. (2012) 'Doxycycline for osteoarthritis of the knee or hip', *Cochrane Database of Systematic Reviews*.

Cramp, F., Hewlett, S., Almeida, C., Kirwan, J., Choy, E., et al. (2013) 'Non-pharmacological interventions for fatigue in rheumatoid arthritis', *Cochrane Database of Systematic Reviews*.

Curtis, J. and Singh, J. (2011) 'Use of biologics in rheumatoid arthritis: current and emerging paradigms of care', *Clinical Therapeutics*, 33(6): 679–707.

Cutolo, M. (2001) 'Anti-inflammatory mechanisms of methotrexate in rheumatoid arthritis', *Annals of the Rheumatic Diseases*, 60(8): 729–35.

Davis, A. and Robson, J. (2016) 'The dangers of NSAIDs: look both ways', *British Journal of General Practice*, 66(645): 172–3.

DAWN (2017) 'HAQ-DI: Health assessment questionnaire'. Available online at: <www.4s-dawn.com/HAQ/HAQ-DI.html>.

De Souza, I. C. C. (2014) 'Pathophysiology and etiology of osteoarthritis'. Available online at: <www.esciencecentral.org/ebooks/osteoarthritis_therapeutics/pathophysiology-and-etiology-of-osteoarthritis.php>.

Dejaco, C., Singh, Y., Perel, P., Hutchings, A., Camellino, D., et al. (2015) '2015 recommendations for the management of polymyalgia rheumatica: A European League Against Rheumatism/American College of Rheumatology Collaborative initiative', *Arthritis & Rheumatology*, 67(10): 2569–80.

Derry, S., Conaghan, P., Da Silva, J., Wiffen, P. and Moore, R. (2016) 'Topical NSAIDs for chronic musculoskeletal pain in adults', *Cochrane Database of Systematic Reviews*.

Ding, D., Lawson, K., Kolbe-Alexander, T., Finkelstein, E., Katzmarzyk, P., et al. (2016) 'The economic burden of physical inactivity: a global analysis of major non-communicable diseases', *The Lancet*, 388(10051): 1311–24.

Duivenvoorden, T., Brouwer, R., van Raaij, T., Verhagen, A., Verhaar, J. and Bierma-Zeinstra, S. (2015) 'Braces and orthoses for treating osteoarthritis of the knee', *Cochrane Database of Systematic Reviews*.

Durme, C. van, Wechalekar, M., Buchbinder, R., Schlesinger, N., van der Heijde, D., et al. (2014) 'Non-steroidal anti-inflammatory drugs for acute gout', *Cochrane Database of Systematic Reviews*.

Eckstein, F., Hudelmaier, M. and Putz, R. (2006) 'The effects of exercise on human articular cartilage', *Journal of Anatomy*, 208(4): 491–512.

Ekelund, U., Steene-Johannessen, J., Brown, W., Fagerland, M., Owen, N., et al. (2016) 'Does physical activity attenuate, or even eliminate, the detrimental association of sitting time with mortality? A harmonised meta-analysis of data from more than 1 million men and women', *The Lancet*, 388(10051): 1302–10.

Eun-Kyoo S., Jae-Young M., Jong-Keun S. and Yim Ji-H. (2013) *The Evolution of Modern Total Knee Prostheses* (1st edn). INTECH Open Access Publisher.

Fernandes, L., Hagen, K., Bijlsma, J., Andreassen, O., Christensen, P., et al. (2013) 'EULAR recommendations for the non-pharmacological core management of hip and knee osteoarthritis', *Annals of the Rheumatic Diseases*, 72(7): 1125–35.

Finckh, A., Escher, M., Liang, M. and Bansback, N. (2016) 'Preventive treatments for rheumatoid arthritis: issues regarding patient preferences', *Current Rheumatology Reports*, 18(8): 51.

Fisher, E., Law, E., Palermo, T. and Eccleston, C. (2015) 'Psychological therapies (remotely delivered) for the management of chronic and recurrent pain in children and adolescents', *Cochrane Database of Systematic Reviews*.

Fransen, M., McConnell, S., Hernandez-Molina, G. and Reichenbach, S. (2014) 'Exercise for osteoarthritis of the hip', *Cochrane Database of Systematic Reviews*.

French, H., Galvin, R., Abbott, J. and Fransen, M. (2015) 'Adjunctive therapies in addition to land-based exercise therapy for osteoarthritis of the hip or knee', *Cochrane Database of Systematic Reviews*.

Garnero, P. (2007) 'New biochemical markers of cartilage turnover in osteoarthritis: Recent developments and remaining challenges', *BoneKEy-Osteovision*, 4(1): 7–18.

Genevay, S. and Atlas, S. (2010) 'Lumbar spinal stenosis', *Best Practice & Research Clinical Rheumatology*, 24(2): 253–65.

Gerlag, D., Norris, J. and Tak, P. (2015) 'Towards prevention of autoantibody-positive rheumatoid arthritis: from lifestyle modification to preventive treatment', *Rheumatology*, 55(4): 607–14.

Glanville, J., Higgens, C. and Mouyis, M. (2016) 'An approach to joint pain and inflammatory arthropathies', *British Journal of Hospital Medicine*, 77(7): C109–C111.

Gonzalez-Gay, M., Garcia-Porrua, C., Miranda-Filloy, J. and Martin, J. (2006) 'Giant cell arteritis and polymyalgia rheumatica', *Drugs & Aging*, 23(8): 627–49.

GPonline (2010) 'Clinical review: Degenerative spine disease'. Available online at: <www.gponline.com/clinical-review-degenerative-spine-disease/musc uloskeletal-disorders/article/1029192>.

Graham, G. and Scott, K. (2005) 'Mechanism of action of paracetamol', *American Journal of Therapeutics*, 12(1): 46–55.

Han, A., Judd, M., Welch, V., Wu, T., Tugwell, P. and Wells, G. (2004) 'Tai chi for treating rheumatoid arthritis', *Cochrane Database of Systematic Reviews*.

Harvard Health (2017) 'Pseudogout (CPPD)'. Available online at: <www. health.harvard.edu/diseases-and-conditions/pseudogout-cppd>.

Hawke, F., Burns, J., Radford, J. and du Toit, V. (2008) 'Custom-made foot orthoses for the treatment of foot pain', *Cochrane Database of Systematic Reviews*.

Heeringa, J. (2005) 'Prevalence, incidence and lifetime risk of atrial fibrillation: the Rotterdam study', *European Heart Journal*, 27(8): 949–53.

Hewlett, S. (2002) 'Measuring the meaning of disability in rheumatoid arthritis: the Personal Impact Health Assessment Questionnaire (PI HAQ)', *Annals of the Rheumatic Diseases*, 61(11): 986–93.

Hoving, J., Lacaille, D., Urquhart, D., Hannu, T., Sluiter, J., et al. (2014) 'Non-pharmacological interventions for preventing job loss in workers with inflammatory arthritis', *Cochrane Database of Systematic Reviews*.

Instant Anatomy (2009) 'Classification of joints'. Available online at: <www.instantanatomy.net/arm/joints/classification.html>.

Jason, M., Highsmith, M., Nicola, V. and Hawkinson, R. (2016) 'Degenerative disc disease center – treatments, symptoms, causes'. Available online at: <www.spineuniverse.com/conditions/degenerative-disc-disease>.

Jobanputra, P. (2003) 'A survey of British rheumatologists' DMARD preferences for rheumatoid arthritis', *Rheumatology*, 43(2): 206–10.

Jüni, P., Hari, R., Rutjes, A., Fischer, R., Silletta, M., et al. (2015) 'Intra-articular corticosteroid for knee osteoarthritis', *Cochrane Database of Systematic Reviews*.

Karsdal, M., Byrjalsen, I., Bay-Jensen, A., Henriksen, K., Riis, B., et al. (2010) 'Biochemical markers identify influences on bone and cartilage degradation in osteoarthritis – the effect of sex, Kellgren-Lawrence (KL) score, Body Mass Index (BMI), oral salmon calcitonin (sCT) treatment and diurnal variation', *BMC Musculoskeletal Disorders*, 11(1): 125.

Kavanaugh, A. (2008) 'Interleukin-6 inhibitors in the treatment of rheumatoid arthritis', *Therapeutics and Clinical Risk Management*, 4: 767–75.

Kennedy, S. (2012) 'Polymyalgia rheumatica and giant cell arteritis: An in-depth look at diagnosis and treatment', *Journal of the American Academy of Nurse Practitioners*, 24(5): 277–85.

Kent, P. and Kjaer, P. (2012) 'The efficacy of targeted interventions for modifiable psychosocial risk factors of persistent nonspecific low back pain – A systematic review', *Manual Therapy*, 17(5): 385–401.

Kidd, B. (2001) 'Mechanisms of inflammatory pain', *British Journal of Anaesthesia*, 87(1): 3–11.

Knight, S., Aujla, R. and Biswas, S. (2011) 'Total hip arthroplasty – over 100 years of operative history', *Orthopedic Reviews*, 3(2): 16.

Knott, L. (2015) 'Calcium pyrophosphate deposition – including pseudogout'. Available online at: <http://patient.info/doctor/ calcium-pyrophosphate-deposition-including-pseudogout-pro>.

Kraan, P. van der, Matta, C. and Mobasheri, A. (2016) 'Age-related altera-tions in signaling pathways in articular chondrocytes: implications for the pathogenesis and progression of osteoarthritis – a mini-review', *Gerontology*, 63(1): 29–35.

Kroon, F., van der Burg, L., Buchbinder, R., Osborne, R., Johnston, R. and Pitt, V. (2014) 'Self-management education programmes for osteoar-thritis', *Cochrane Database of Systematic Reviews*.

Kroon, F., van der Burg, L., Ramiro, S., Landewé, R., Buchbinder, R., et al. (2015) 'Non-steroidal anti-inflammatory drugs (NSAIDs) for axial spondyloarthritis (ankylosing spondylitis and non-radiographic axial spondyloarthritis)', *Cochrane Database of Systematic Reviews*.

Kuettner, K. and Cole, A. (2005) 'Cartilage degeneration in different human joints', *Osteoarthritis and Cartilage*, 13(2): 93–103.

Kuijpers, T., van Middelkoop, M., Rubinstein, S., Ostelo, R., Verhagen, A., et al. (2010) 'A systematic review on the effectiveness of pharmacological interventions for chronic non-specific low-back pain', *European Spine Journal*, 20(1): 40–50.

Kydd, A., Seth, R., Buchbinder, R., Edwards, C. and Bombardier, C. (2014) 'Uricosuric medications for chronic gout', *Cochrane Database of Systematic Reviews*.

Lab Tests Online (2016) 'Septic arthritis'. Available online at: <http://labtestsonline.org.uk/understanding/conditions/septic/>.

Lab Tests Online (2017) 'Arthritis'. Available online at: <http://labtestson-line.org.uk/understanding/conditions/arthritis/>.

Lab Tests Online (2017) 'Gout'. Available online at: <http://labtestsonline.org.uk/understanding/conditions/gout>.

Lab Tests Online (2017) 'Osteoarthritis'. Available online at: <http://labtest-sonline.org.uk/understanding/conditions/osteo>.

Lahiri, M., Morgan, C., Symmons, D. and Bruce, I. (2011) 'Modifiable risk factors for RA: prevention, better than cure?', *Rheumatology*, 51(3): 499–512.

Lee, A., Ellman, M., Yan, D., Kroin, J., Cole, B., et al. (2013) 'A current review of molecular mechanisms regarding osteoarthritis and pain', *Gene*, 527(2): 440–7.

Li, S., Yu, B., Zhou, D., He, C., Zhuo, Q. and Hulme, J. (2013) 'Electromagnetic fields for treating osteoarthritis', *Cochrane Database of Systematic Reviews*.

Liddle, S. and Pennick, V. (2015) 'Interventions for preventing and treating low-back and pelvic pain during pregnancy', *Cochrane Database of Systematic Reviews*.

Livshits, G., Ermakov, S. and Vilker, A. (2010) 'Outlines of the biochemistry of osteoarthritis', *Current Rheumatology Reviews*, 6(4): 234–50.

Lotz, M., Martel-Pelletier, J., Christiansen, C., Brandi, M., Bruyère, O., et al. (2013) 'Value of biomarkers in osteoarthritis: current status and perspec-tives', *Annals of the Rheumatic Diseases*, 72(11): 1756–63.

McAlindon, T., Bannuru, R., Sullivan, M., Arden, N., Berenbaum, F., et al. (2014) 'OARSI guidelines for the non-surgical management of knee osteoarthritis', *Osteoarthritis and Cartilage*, 22(3): 363–88.

Malfait, A. and Schnitzer, T. (2013) 'Towards a mechanism-based approach to pain management in osteoarthritis', *Nature Reviews Rheumatology*, 9(11): 654–64.

Manheimer, E., Cheng, K., Linde, K., Lao, L., Yoo, J., et al. (2010) 'Acupuncture for peripheral joint osteoarthritis', *Cochrane Database of Systematic Reviews*.

Maniadakis, N. and Gray, A. (2000) 'The economic burden of back pain in the UK', *Pain*, 84(1): 95–103.

Marks, J., Colebatch, A., Buchbinder, R. and Edwards, C. (2011) 'Pain management for rheumatoid arthritis and cardiovascular or renal comorbidity', *Cochrane Database of Systematic Reviews*.

Mayo Clinic (2016) 'Bursitis'. Available online at: <www.mayoclinic.org/diseases-conditions/bursitis/basics/definition/con-20015102>.

Md Yusof, M. and Emery, P. (2013) 'Targeting interleukin-6 in rheumatoid arthritis', *Drugs*, 73(4): 341–56.

Medscape (2016) 'Fibromyalgia: practice essentials, background, pathophysiology'. Available online at: <http://emedicine.medscape.com/article/329838-overview#a2>.

Medscape (2016) 'Osteoarthritis: practice essentials, background, anatomy'. Available online at: <http://emedicine.medscape.com/article/330487-overview#a5>.

Mifflin, K. and Kerr, B. (2016) 'Pain in autoimmune disorders', *Journal of Neuroscience Research*, 95: 1282–94.

Mobasheri, A. and Batt, M. (2016) 'An update on the pathophysiology of osteoarthritis', *Annals of Physical and Rehabilitation Medicine*, 59(5–6): 333–9.

Moore, R., Wiffen, P., Derry, S., Maguire, T., Roy, Y. and Tyrrell, L. (2015) 'Non-prescription (OTC) oral analgesics for acute pain – an overview of Cochrane reviews', *Cochrane Database of Systematic Reviews*.

MSD Manual Professional Edition (2017) 'Osteoarthritis (OA) – musculoskeletal and connective tissue disorders'. Available online at: <www.msdmanuals.com/en-gb/professional/musculoskeletal-and-connective-tissue-disorders/joint-disorders/osteoarthritis-oa>.

Nagai, M., Ito, A., Tajino, J., Iijima, H., Yamaguchi, S., et al. (2016) 'Remobilization causes site-specific cyst formation in immobilization-induced knee cartilage degeneration in an immobilized rat model', *Journal of Anatomy*, 228(6): 929–39.

NASS (2017) 'Clinical guidelines'. Available online at: <www.spine.org/ResearchClinicalCare/QualityImprovement/ClinicalGuidelines.aspx>.

NASS (2017) 'Resources for health professionals'. Available online at: <http://nass.co.uk/healthcare-professionals/resources-for-health-professionals/>.

National Institute of Arthritis and Musculoskeletal and Skin Diseases (2017) 'Questions and answers about reactive arthritis'. Available online at: <www.niams.nih.gov/health_info/Reactive_Arthritis/>.

National Joint Registry (2017) 'ReportsOnline'. Available online at: <www.njrcentre.org.uk/njrcentre/Healthcareproviders/Accessingthedata/ReportsOnline/tabid/118/Default.aspx>.

National Rheumatoid Arthritis Society (2017) 'Anti-TNFa treatment in rheumatoid arthritis'. Available online at: <www.nras.org.uk/anti-tnfa-treatment-in-rheumatoid-arthritis>.

National Rheumatoid Arthritis Society (2017) 'Immunisation for people with rheumatoid arthritis'. Available online at: <www.nras.org.uk/immunisation-for-people-with-rheumatoid-arthritis->.

National Rheumatoid Arthritis Society (2017) 'The DAS28 score'. Available online at: <www.nras.org.uk/the-das28-score>.

Nature (2017) 'Rheumatoid arthritis – Latest research and news'. Available online at: <www.nature.com/subjects/rheumatoid-arthritis>.

NCCIH (2016) 'Osteoarthritis: in depth'. Available online at: <https://nccih. nih.gov/health/arthritis/osteoarthritis#hed3>.

NICE (2009) 'Individually magnetic resonance imaging-designed unicompartmental interpositional implant insertion for osteoarthritis of the knee'. Available online at: <www.nice.org.uk/guidance/ipg317>.

NICE (2013) 'Ankylosing spondylitis'. Available online at: <https://cks.nice. org.uk/ankylosing-spondylitis#!evidence>.

NICE (2013) 'Polymyalgia rheumatica'. Available online at: <https://cks. nice.org.uk/polymyalgia-rheumatica#!backgroundsub:2>.

NICE (2013) 'Rheumatoid arthritis'. Available online at: <https://cks.nice. org.uk/rheumatoid-arthritis#!diagnosissub:2>.

NICE (2014) 'Osteoarthritis: care and management'. Available online at: <www.nice.org.uk/guidance/cg177>.

NICE (2014) 'Platelet-rich plasma injections for osteoarthritis of the knee'. Available online at: <www.nice.org.uk/guidance/ipg491>.

NICE (2015) 'Implantation of a shock or load absorber for mild to moderate symptomatic medial knee osteoarthritis'. Available online at: <www. nice.org.uk/guidance/ipg512>.

NICE (2015) 'Joint distraction for ankle osteoarthritis'. Available online at: <www.nice.org.uk/guidance/ipg538>.

NICE (2015) 'Joint distraction for knee osteoarthritis without alignment correction'. Available online at: <www.nice.org.uk/guidance/ipg529>.

NICE (2015) 'Osteoarthritis'. Available online at: <https://cks.nice.org.uk/ osteoarthritis#!backgroundsub:1>.

NICE (2016) 'Osteoarthritis: care and management'. Available online at: <www. nice.org.uk/guidance/cg177/chapter/1-Recommendations#referral-for-consideration-of-joint-surgery-2>.

NICE (2016) 'Rheumatoid arthritis in adults: management'. Available online at: <www.nice.org.uk/guidance/cg79/chapter/Recommendations #pharmacological-management>.

NICE (2017) 'Ankylosing spondylitis'. Available online at: <https://cks.nice. org.uk/ankylosing-spondylitis#!scenariorecommendation:4>.

NICE (2017) 'DMARDs'. Available online at: <https://cks.nice.org.uk/ dmards#!scenario>.

Oltean, H., Robbins, C., van Tulder, M., Berman, B., Bombardier, C., et al. (2014) 'Herbal medicine for low-back pain', *Cochrane Database of Systematic Reviews*.

Omoigui, S. (2007) 'The biochemical origin of pain: The origin of all pain is inflammation and the inflammatory response, Part 2 of 3 – Inflammatory profile of pain syndromes'. *Medical Hypotheses*, 69(6): 1169–78.

Osterweis, M., Kleinman, A. and Mechanic, D. (1988) *Pain and Disability* (1st edn). Washington, DC: National Academy Press.

OzRadOnc (2017) '7.3 – Principles of MRI scanning'. Available online at: <http://ozradonc.wikidot.com/principles-of-mri-scanning>.

Palmer, J., Monk, A., Hopewell, S., Bayliss, L., Jackson, W., et al. (2016)

'Surgical interventions for early structural knee osteoarthritis', *Cochrane Database of Systematic Reviews*.

Patient Info (2016) 'Spinal disc problems (including red flag signs) information'. Available online at: <http://patient.info/doctor/spinal-disc-problems-including-red-flag-signs>.

Pergolizzi, J., Ahlbeck, K., Aldington, D., Alon, E., Coluzzi, F., et al. (2013) 'The development of chronic pain: physiological CHANGE necessitates a multidisciplinary approach to treatment', *Current Medical Research and Opinion*, 29(9): 1127–35.

Perioperative Pain (2001) 'Neuroanatomy of pain'. Available online at: <www.perioperativepain.com/Neuroanatomy_of_Pain.htm>.

Plotnikoff, R., Karunamuni, N., Lytvyak, E., Penfold, C., Schopflocher, D., et al. (2015) 'Osteoarthritis prevalence and modifiable factors: a population study', *BMC Public Health*, 15(1): 1195.

Poquet, N., Lin, C., Heymans, M., van Tulder, M., Esmail, R., et al. (2016) 'Back schools for acute and subacute non-specific low-back pain', *Cochrane Database of Systematic Reviews*.

Punchard, N., Greenfield, S. and Thompson, R. (1992) 'Mechanism of action of 5-aminosalicylic acid', *Mediators of Inflammation*, 1(3): 151–65.

Ramiro, S., Radner, H., van der Heijde, D., van Tubergen, A., Buchbinder, R., et al. (2011) 'Combination therapy for pain management in inflammatory arthritis (rheumatoid arthritis, ankylosing spondylitis, psoriatic arthritis, other spondyloarthritis)', *Cochrane Database of Systematic Reviews*.

Regnaux, J., Lefevre-Colau, M., Trinquart, L., Nguyen, C., Boutron, I., et al. (2015) 'High-intensity versus low-intensity physical activity or exercise in people with hip or knee osteoarthritis', *Cochrane Database of Systematic Reviews*.

RheumaKit (2017) 'DAS28 calculator'. Available online at: <www.rheumakit.com/en/calculators/das28>.

Richards, B., Whittle, S. and Buchbinder, R. (2011) 'Antidepressants for pain management in rheumatoid arthritis', *Cochrane Database of Systematic Reviews*.

Richards, B., Whittle, S. and Buchbinder, R. (2012) 'Muscle relaxants for pain management in rheumatoid arthritis', *Cochrane Database of Systematic Reviews*.

Richards, B., Whittle, S. and Buchbinder, R. (2012) 'Neuromodulators for pain management in rheumatoid arthritis', *Cochrane Database of Systematic Reviews*.

Rituxan, R. A. (2017) 'Important safety information'. Available online at: <www.rituxanforra-hcp.com/isi>.

Rituxan, R. A. (2017) 'Infusion-related adverse reactions'. Available online at: <www.rituxanforra-hcp.com/safety/infusion-reactions>.

Rooij, M. de, van der Leeden, M., Cheung, J., van der Esch, M., Häkkinen, A., et al. (2016) 'Efficacy of tailored exercise therapy on physical functioning in patients with knee osteoarthritis and comorbidity: A randomized controlled trial', *Arthritis Care & Research*, doi:10.1002/acr.23013.

Rothschild, B. (2011) 'Contributions of paleorheumatology to understanding contemporary disease', *Reumatismo*, 54(3): 272–84.

Rothschild, B. M. and Woods, R. J. (2012) *Epidemiology and Biomechanics of Osteoarthritis* (1st edn). INTECH Open Access Publisher.

Salisbury NHS Foundation Trust (2017) 'Septic arthritis antibiotic guidance'. Available online at: <www.icid.salisbury.nhs.uk/MedicinesManagement/Guidance/AntimicrobialMedicine/Pages/SepticArthritisAntibioticGuidance.aspx>.

Saragiotto, B., Machado, G., Ferreira, M., Pinheiro, M., Abdel Shaheed, C. et al. (2016) 'Paracetamol for low back pain', *Cochrane Database of Systematic Reviews*.

Schlesinger, N. and Schlesinger, M. (2013) 'Previously reported prior studies of cherry juice concentrate for gout flare prophylaxis: Comment on the article by Zhang et al', *Arthritis & Rheumatism*, 65(4): 1135–6.

Scott, D., Wolfe, F. and Huizinga, T. (2010) 'Rheumatoid arthritis', *The Lancet*, 376(9746): 1094–108.

Seth, R., Kydd, A., Buchbinder, R., Bombardier, C. and Edwards, C. (2014) 'Allopurinol for chronic gout', *Cochrane Database of Systematic Reviews*.

Shea, B., Swinden, M., Tanjong Ghogomu, E., Ortiz, Z., Katchamart, W., et al. (2013) 'Folic acid and folinic acid for reducing side effects in patients receiving methotrexate for rheumatoid arthritis', *Cochrane Database of Systematic Reviews*.

Shea, B., Swinden, M., Tanjong Ghogomu, E., Ortiz, Z., Katchamart, W., et al. (2013) 'Folic acid and folinic acid for reducing side effects in patients receiving methotrexate for rheumatoid arthritis', *Cochrane Database of Systematic Reviews*.

Shemory, S., Pfefferle, K. and Gradisar, I. (2016) 'Modifiable risk factors in patients with low back pain', *Orthopedics*, 39(3): e413–e416.

Shiel, W. Jr., (2017) 'Is it possible to prevent polymyalgia rheumatica?' Available online at: <www.medicinenet.com/polymyalgia_rheumatica/page3.htm>.

Sieper, J. (2001) 'Pathogenesis of reactive arthritis', *Current Rheumatology Reports*, 3(5): 412–18.

Simanek, V., Kren, V., Ulrichova, J. and Gallo, J. (2005) 'The efficacy of glucosamine and chondroitin sulfate in the treatment of osteoarthritis: are these saccharides drugs or nutraceuticals?', *Biomedical Papers*, 149(1): 51–6.

Singh, J., Bharat, A. and Edwards, N. (2015) 'An internet survey of common treatments used by patients with gout including cherry extract and juice and other dietary supplements', *Journal of Clinical Rheumatology*, 21(4): 225–6.

Singh, J., Christensen, R., Wells, G., Suarez-Almazor, M., Buchbinder, R., et al. (2009) 'Biologics for rheumatoid arthritis: an overview of Cochrane reviews', *Cochrane Database of Systematic Reviews*.

Singh, J., Sperling, J., Buchbinder, R. and McMaken, K. (2010) 'Surgery for shoulder osteoarthritis', *Cochrane Database of Systematic Reviews*.

Smith, C. and Grimmer-Somers, K. (2010) 'The treatment effect of exercise programmes for chronic low back pain', *Journal of Evaluation in Clinical Practice*, 16(3): 484–91.

Smith, M. D. (2011) 'The normal synovium', *The Open Rheumatology Journal*, 5(1): 100–6.

Steultjens, E., Dekker, J., Bouter, L., Schaardenburg, D., Kuyk, M., et al. (2004) 'Occupational therapy for rheumatoid arthritis', *Cochrane Database of Systematic Reviews*.

Straube, S., Derry, S., Straube, C. and Moore, R. (2015) 'Vitamin D for the treatment of chronic painful conditions in adults', *Cochrane Database of Systematic Reviews*.

Sulsky, S., Carlton, L., Bochmann, F., Ellegast, R., Glitsch, U., et al. (2012) 'Epidemiological evidence for work load as a risk factor for osteoarthritis of the hip: a systematic review', *PLoS ONE*, 7(2): e31521.

Suokas, A., Walsh, D., McWilliams, D., Condon, L., Moreton, B., et al. (2012) 'Quantitative sensory testing in painful osteoarthritis: a systematic review and meta-analysis', *Osteoarthritis and Cartilage*, 20(10): 1075–85.

Tanaka, Y. and Martin Mola, E. (2014) 'IL-6 targeting compared to TNF targeting in rheumatoid arthritis: studies of olokizumab, sarilumab and sirukumab', *Annals of the Rheumatic Diseases*, 73(9): 1595–7.

TeachMeAnatomy (2017) 'The wrist joint'. Available online at: <http://teachmeanatomy.info/upper-limb/joints/wrist-joint/>.

Thysen, S., Luyten, F. and Lories, R. (2015) 'Targets, models and challenges in osteoarthritis research', *Disease Models & Mechanisms*, 8(1): 17–30.

Toivanen, A. (2000) 'Managing reactive arthritis', *Rheumatology*, 39(2): 117–19.

Toupet, K., Maumus, M., Peyrafitte, J., Bourin, P., Jorgensen, C., et al. (2012) 'Long-term detection of human adipose tissue-derived mesenchymal stem cells after intra-articular injection', *Osteoarthritis and Cartilage*, 20: S51–S52.

Tzortziou Brown, V., Underwood, M., Mohamed, N., Westwood, O. and Morrissey, D. (2016) 'Professional interventions for general practitioners on the management of musculoskeletal conditions', *Cochrane Database of Systematic Reviews*.

University of Wisconsin School of Medicine and Public Health (2010) 'Basic definitions & clinical implications – pain management'. Available online at: <http://projects.hsl.wisc.edu/GME/PainManagement/session 2.1.html>.

Verhagen, A., Bierma-Zeinstra, S., Boers, M., Cardoso, J., Lambeck, J., et al. (2015) 'Balneotherapy (or spa therapy) for rheumatoid arthritis', *Cochrane Database of Systematic Reviews*.

Vierck, C. (2012) 'A mechanism-based approach to prevention of and therapy for fibromyalgia', *Pain Research and Treatment*, 2012: 1–12.

Vincent, K., Conrad, B., Fregly, B. and Vincent, H. (2012) 'The pathophysiology of osteoarthritis: a mechanical perspective on the knee joint', *PM&R*, 4(5): S–S9.

Vindigni, D., Walker, B., Jamison, J., Da Costa, C., Parkinson, L. et al. (2005) 'Low back pain risk factors in a large rural Australian Aboriginal community: An opportunity for managing co-morbidities', *Chiropractic & Osteopathy*, 13(1): 21.

Vivek Sood, M (2014) 'Cemented vs. cementless alternatives in joint replacement'. Arthritis Health. Available online at: <www.arthritis-health.com/surgery/type/cemented-vs-cementless-alternatives-joint-replacement>.

Wallen, M. and Gillies, D. (2006) 'Intra-articular steroids and splints/rest for children with juvenile idiopathic arthritis and adults with rheumatoid arthritis', *Cochrane Database of Systematic Reviews*.

Wang, X., Hunter, D., Xu, J. and Ding, C. (2015) 'Metabolic triggered inflammation in osteoarthritis', *Osteoarthritis and Cartilage*, 23(1): 22–30.

WebMD (2016) 'Fibromyalgia tender points and trigger points'. Available online at: <www.webmd.com/fibromyalgia/guide/fibromyalgia-tender-points-trigger-points>.

WebMD (2017) 'Lumbar spinal stenosis – prevention'. Available online at: <www.webmd.com/back-pain/tc/lumbar-spinal-stenosis-prevention>.

Whittaker, R. (2015) 'Classification of joints', Instant Anatomy. Available online at: <www.instantanatomy.net/arm/joints/classification.html>.

Whittle, S., Richards, B., Husni, E. and Buchbinder, R. (2011) 'Opioid therapy for treating rheumatoid arthritis pain', *Cochrane Database of Systematic Reviews*.

Wilke, W. (2009) 'Fibromyalgia', Cleveland Clinic Centre for Continuing Education. Available online at: <www.clevelandclinicmeded.com/medical pubs/diseasemanagement/rheumatology/fibromyalgia-syndrome/>.

Williams, D. and Gracely, R. (2006) 'Biology and therapy of fibromyalgia: Functional magnetic resonance imaging findings in fibromyalgia', *Arthritis Research & Therapy*, 8(6): 224.

Witrouw, E. and Van Ginckel, A. (2015) 'Effects of exercise on cartilage status', *Aspetar Sports Medicine Journal*. Available online at: <www.aspetar.com/journal/viewarticle.aspx?id=97#.V9GH4lsrJdg>.

Witteveen, A., Hofstad, C. and Kerkhoffs, G. (2015) 'Hyaluronic acid and other conservative treatment options for osteoarthritis of the ankle', *Cochrane Database of Systematic Reviews*.

Yalçın, S., Kara, M., Öztürk, G. and Özçakar, L. (2016) 'Ultrasonographic measurements of the metacarpal and talar cartilage thicknesses in hemiplegic patients after stroke', *Topics in Stroke Rehabilitation*, 24(1): 1–4.

Yang, N. and Meng, Q. (2016) 'Circadian clocks in articular cartilage and bone', *Journal of Biological Rhythms*, 31(5): 415–27.

Zhang, W., Doherty, M., Pascual, E., Barskova, V., Guerne, P., et al. (2011) 'EULAR recommendations for calcium pyrophosphate deposition, Part II: Management'. *Annals of the Rheumatic Diseases*, 70(4): 571–5.

Zhang, W., Ouyang, H., Dass, C. and Xu, J. (2016) 'Current research on pharmacologic and regenerative therapies for osteoarthritis', *Bone Research*, 4, 15040.

Zhang, Y., Neogi, T., Chen, C., Chaisson, C., Hunter, D. and Choi, H. (2012) 'Cherry consumption and decreased risk of recurrent gout attacks', *Arthritis & Rheumatism*, 64(12): 4004–11.

Zochling, J. (2006) 'Current evidence for the management of ankylosing spondylitis: a systematic literature review for the ASAS/EULAR management recommendations in ankylosing spondylitis', *Annals of the Rheumatic Diseases*, 65(4): 423–32.

Zupan, J., Jeras, M. and Marc, J. (2013) 'Osteoimmunology and the influence of pro-inflammatory cytokines on osteoclasts', *Biochemia Medica* 23(1): 43–63.

Index